IT'S ALL GOOD

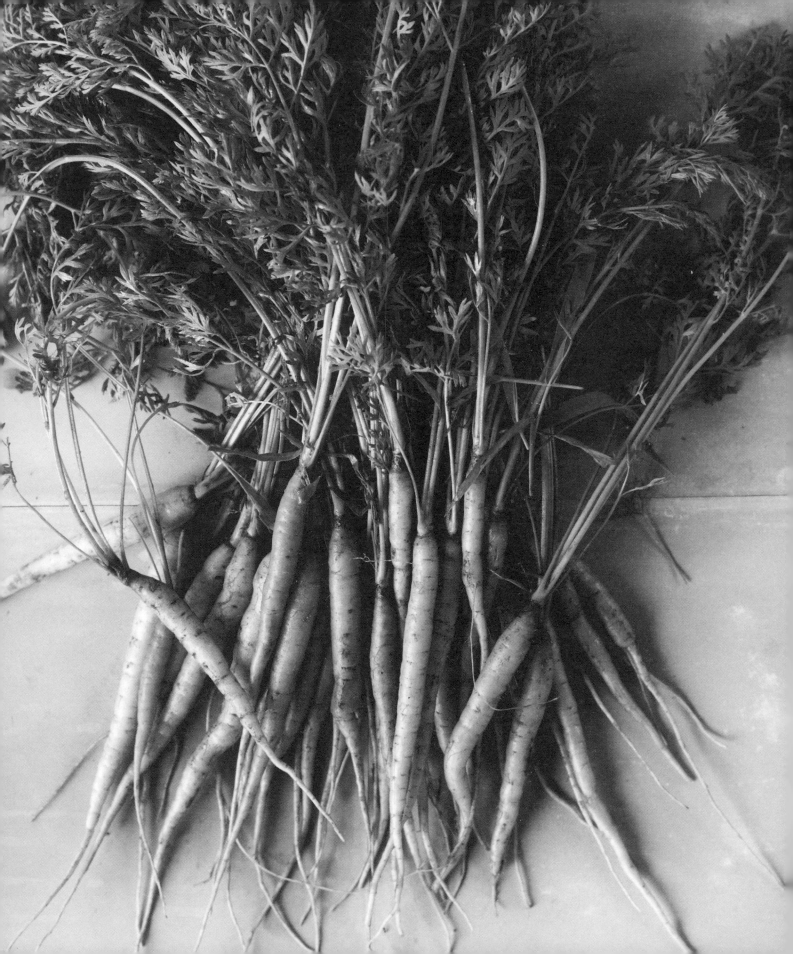

IT'S ALL GOOD

Delicious, Easy Recipes That Will Make You Look Good and Feel Great

Gwyneth Paltrow

and Julia Turshen

Photographs by Ditte Isager

sphere

SPHERE

This paperback edition published in 2013 by Sphere
Reprinted 2013

First published in the United States of America in 2013 by Grand Central

The moral right of the author has been asserted.

A CIP catalogue record for this book
is available from the British Library.

ISBN 978-0-3494-0083-9

Printed and bound in Italy

Sphere
An imprint of
Little, Brown Book Group
100 Victoria Embankment
London EC4Y 0DY

An Hachette UK Company
www.hachette.co.uk

www.littlebrown.co.uk

I dedicate this book to the amazing men and women who have
taught me that food is medicine, that consciousness
is everything, that a clean body makes a happy existence,
and that how you relate to the issue is the issue!—
Dr. Habib Sadeghi, Dr. Alejandro Junger, Michio Kushi,
John Kenyon, Janet Reibstein, Vicky Vlachonis,
and Lee and Darleen Gross.

• • •

For Chris, Apple, and Moses.
For Whistler.

— Gwyneth

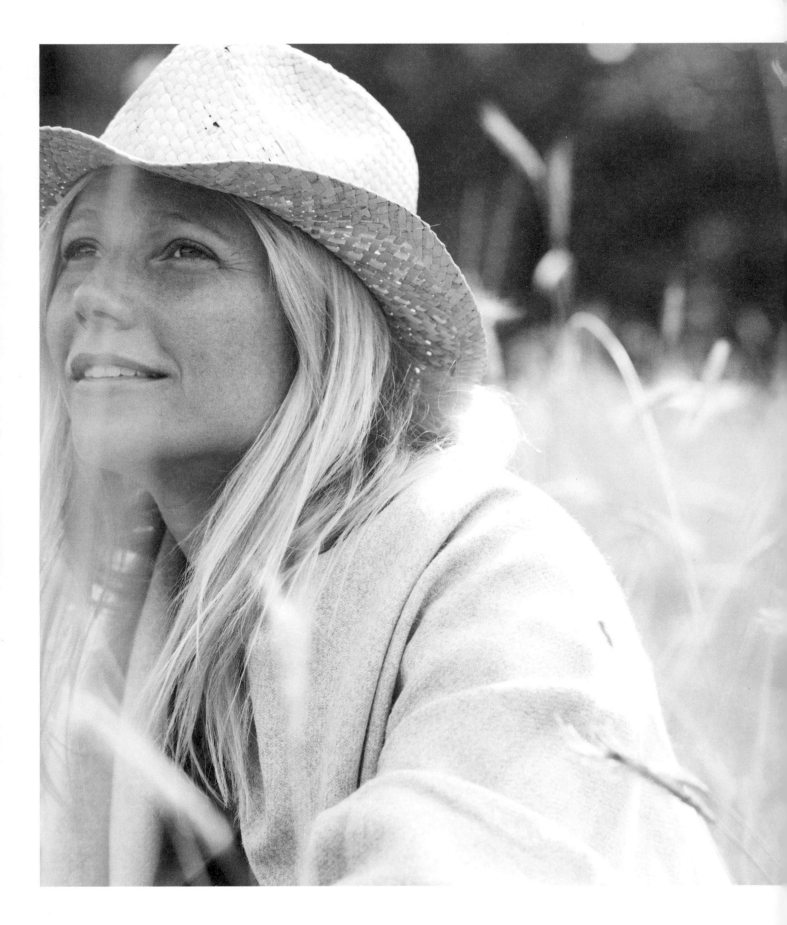

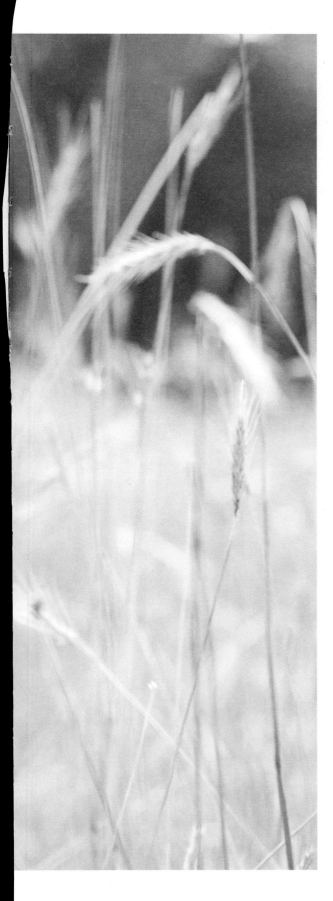

Contents

Foreword

By Dr. Habib Sadeghi

Osteopathic Physician
Be Hive of Healing Center for Integrative Medicine
Los Angeles, California

Food is many things. It's necessary, nurturing, and healing. With few exceptions, food has been misrepresented and sensationalized more than almost any other subject in the media. It seems as though we can't turn on the evening news without seeing a story about a particular food item that was once deemed "bad" for us by an "expert" that's now being praised as healthy.

People are passionate about food. We should be. What's more important than the quality of food that gives us life, health, and strength? Instead of using that passion to enjoy food, we do what we do with most things in life. We complicate it. We overthink it. We worry about whether or not a certain food is good for us, or whether or not it causes some health problem. We've intellectualized food when it's not a mental exercise. It's a sensorial experience. Food comes from the earth. So do we. The tastes, textures, smells, and colors of food are reminders of our visceral connection to the essential life energy of the earth. Food also keeps us aware that we're partners in a process that's much larger than ourselves. Food gives us its life force. In return, we act as good stewards of the earth to ensure this cycle of life continues in a healthy, vital way. We sustain and nurture each other.

Food is simple. Food is spiritual. To understand this, all we need to do is look at the process through which we obtain food's energy: digestion. *Di* means "two" and *gestion* (as in *gestation*) refers to the action of carrying or bearing. Food carries two purposes for us. It has two functions. Everyone understands how food builds and feeds our bodies. When we move away from our instinct and intellectualize food with too much science, we forget that it was created to feed our soul, as well. It builds our bodies through sustenance and nurtures our souls through sensation.

Food is sacred. Its dual purpose was understood by many ancient cultures, which is why food was an integral part of their spiritual ceremonies. The harvest season was celebrated and fertility rituals often included different foods. For thousands of years, Ayurveda, the ancient system of Hindu medicine, has used the energetics of different foods to engage the mind/body connection and facilitate healing. Food isn't an inanimate object. It's part of us. The most intimate way we become one with the earth is by taking what it offers us into our bodies as food. It's a sacred union that's connected to both our divinity as spiritual beings and our human experience through health and vitality.

Food that has fantastic texture, depth of flavor, and an enticing aroma excites us and makes us happy. It thrills us, lights us up, and reminds us what it feels like to enjoy something from the soul level. The experience is even richer when we share food we love with friends and family. It brings us together and strengthens the spiritual connections we have with each

other. We feed our bodies through food, but we feed our souls through what makes us happy, through pleasure. Because food brings us so much pleasure, it's not just essential for a healthy body, but a healthy spirit, too.

A lot of people think great flavor is an afterthought when it comes to "healthy" food, but if we are to be fully nourished by food, it needs to taste wonderful. Food must be a pleasure-filled, spiritual experience. God gave us taste buds for a reason! Animals regularly fed a diet that's full of nutrition but void of any flavor will eventually die from malnutrition.* It's clear that there is a physiological link between taste and health. If we don't enjoy the food we're eating, regardless of whether it's broccoli or brownies, we're absorbing fewer of its nutrients. In order to be fully nourished by our food, we must take pleasure in it.

It seems more than coincidence that my dear friend Gwyneth celebrates her fortieth birthday with the release of this beautiful cookbook. The number forty is highly significant across all traditional faiths and esoteric philosophies. It symbolizes change—coming through a struggle and emerging on the other side more enlightened because of the experience. It's a passage into spiritual adulthood. Traditionally, anyone under the age of forty was prohibited from studying the Jewish mystic philosophy of Kabbalah because it was felt they hadn't had enough life experience to fully digest it. Reaching forty is a joyful milestone. It's a time to celebrate the birth of the new self that has been gestating within. It's time to rejoice in the birth of the body *and* in the rebirth of the soul!

When it comes to cooking amazing food, we all know someone who can come home from work and whip up an incredible meal out of what's left in their refrigerator—usually celery, one egg, sea salt, and three other ingredients that just don't seem to go together. Out of these isolated ingredients comes a terrific meal that makes perfect sense and tastes great. Food is spiritual because it can be a metaphor for life. When crazy things happen and our laundry list of problems just doesn't make sense, we can step back and get a better view of how it's all coming together. We can see how the ingredients complement each other and combine to create a deeper, richer experience. There are no bad ingredients in the recipe of life. Everything adds flavor to the final product and helps us absorb what I call psychospiritual nutrition. We can fully digest all the ingredients of our life and see that they've come together perfectly to make for a fuller human experience. In food and life, **it's all good.**

Dr. Habib Sadeghi
Los Angeles
2012
*David, Marc. *Nourishing Wisdom: A Mind-Body Approach to Nutrition and Well-Being.* New York: Crown Publishing Group, 1994.

On Cooking, Panic Attacks, and Somatization*

One sunny afternoon in London, in the spring of 2011, I thought—without sounding overly dramatic—that I was going to die. I had just served lunch in the garden at home. I had felt unwell while I was preparing it, but I couldn't pinpoint why. I had a vague feeling that I was going to faint, and I wasn't forming thoughts correctly. I didn't say much while we all ate. My family had friends joining us, and it was a beautiful, warm Sunday, but I couldn't really take it in. I was worried. I stood up to clear the table and found that my right hand wasn't working as it should, and then everything went blurry. I got a searing pain in my head, I couldn't speak, and I felt as if I couldn't breathe. I thought I was having a stroke.

My girlfriend held my hand and talked me into a calm state. As it turned out, I was having a horrible migraine and a panic attack. It took me hours to get my equilibrium back. As I tried to sleep it off, I could hear my children playing in the garden, and I was struck by the fear that my health could separate me from them, even for an afternoon. That next week, I set off to see doctors for every imaginable kind of checkup. I was told I had a benign cyst on my ovary that needed to be removed immediately, that I had a nodule on my parathyroid that was causing a lot of my fatigue, that my thyroid wasn't functioning properly, and that I needed to adjust my hormones with more hormones. It was not a good picture.

I had had a very exciting and busy year, and I knew I was worn down from the plane rides, the adrenaline, and the stress. But I didn't realize how this intense period of continuously pressing the override button on my already exhausted system, coupled with lots of French fries and wine, had taken a toll on me. Not to mention these rather serious-sounding physical manifestations of all the stress. I needed to do something. It was time for real change.

* The unfortunate art of turning unexpressed emotion into physical symptoms.

I had always been into health kicks and cleanses and the idea of "being healthy" for the most part, but I usually interspersed this clean living with hearty chunks of happy indulgence. And clearly I had gotten out of balance. I decided I needed to do something to build myself back up, and off I went to see my doctor and good friend Dr. Alejandro Junger. He had blood drawn for many tests, and when he called me a few days later to discuss the results, he sounded surprised. In addition to what had been found in London, I was severely anemic, I was vitamin D deficient, my liver was very congested, my stress levels were sky-high (something about my adrenals), there was a lot of inflammation in my system, and my hormones were off.

Dr. Junger said I needed to go on an elimination diet to clear out my system, heal my gut, and revive my body with good nutrients. This meant no coffee, no alcohol, no dairy, no eggs, no sugar, no shellfish, no deepwater fish, no potatoes, no tomatoes, no bell pepper, no eggplant, no corn, no wheat, no meat, no soy, nothing processed at all—tough words for a foodie to hear. Although it was difficult and I was often stumped about what to eat, I followed the diet to the letter, and three weeks later, I was a different person, according to my blood work. Thrilled that I had accomplished the mission, I asked Dr. Junger when I could go off this incredibly strict diet. "Well, it's hard for me to tell you this because I don't do it myself all the time," he said, "but this is the way you should try to eat for the rest of your life."

The rest of my life? Without Parmesan cheese and fried zucchini and pasta and baguettes and Pinot Noir? I could understand it for a limited time, but always? That was not going to happen, let's face it. However, could it become my baseline? The way I would eat most days, with the occasional cheat day? Could I lean toward it more? I decided I could. I could certainly try. And in the past couple of years, this has become the way I strive to eat and the diet I go back to and adhere to strictly when I have been overindulging, when I need to rebuild or clean out.

That spring in London (when my health and well-being came sharply into focus) became a very important time in my kitchen for my family's health. As I started to focus on eating a very clean, very healthy (sometimes ascetic-feeling) diet, I wondered if it would be possible to make dishes that fit all my new guidelines but tasted, looked, and smelled like the food I usually make. Comfort food with a very healthy bent. Very healthy food that didn't make me feel as if I was missing anything (except the glass of wine!). So I decided to call up my old pal Julia Turshen.

I met Julia during the filming of a food documentary series I did with Mario Batali in 2007 called *Spain…On the Road Again*. Julia was all smiles and all curls and all enthusiasm for food, and before the end of the shoot, we had become fast friends. I asked her what she did when she wasn't at far-flung locations and she said she cooked for a family in New York. In the following months, I found myself in NYC with my family for a week, working hard and unable to prepare our meals. I had an idea: I would ask Julia if she was available to step in. It was the beginning of a beautiful friendship and an incredible collaboration. We realized we loved to cook together, and that the sum of our parts was pretty great. I started to talk to her about an idea I had been thinking over for a long time, a cookbook, *My Father's Daughter*. Julia became my assistant in the

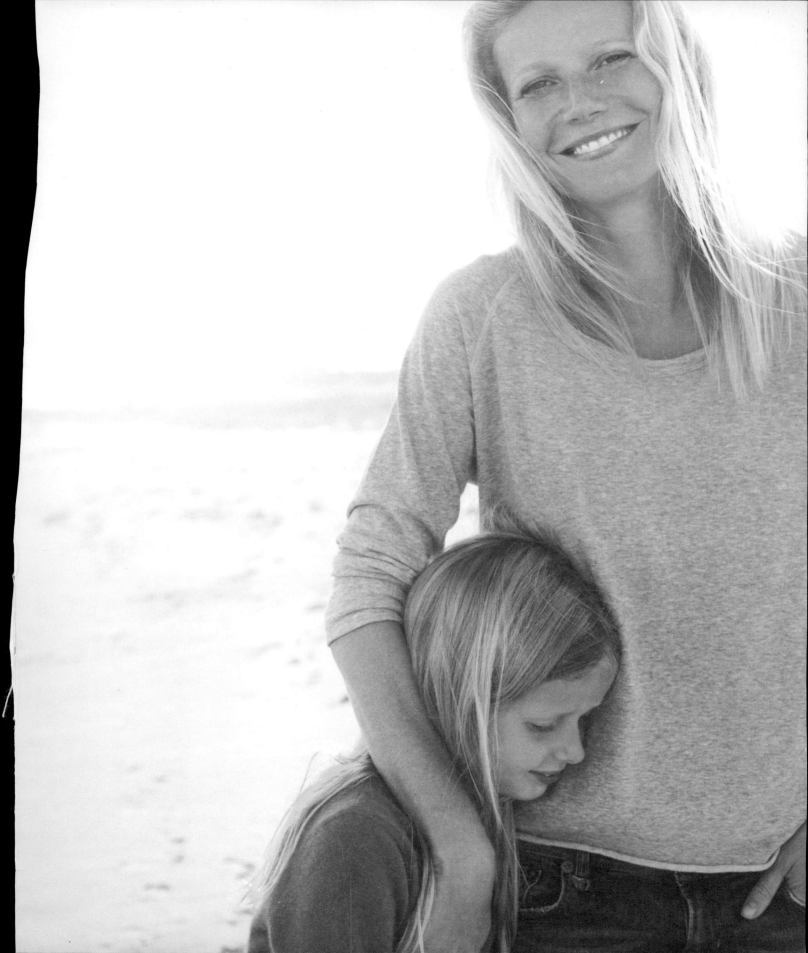

kitchen, and the rest is history. She was my biggest support while I created every recipe for *My Father's Daughter*, standing over my shoulder, taking notes, approximating amounts, and being the best company ever while I worked.

When it was time to think about my next book, I knew I wanted to do it with Julia, but not as my assistant, as my coauthor. We decided to develop all the recipes together this time, bringing that greater-than-the-sum-of-the-parts magic to its utmost manifestation, and having the best f*@£ing time doing it. When thinking of ways to make super-healthy comfort food, inspiration and collaboration were more important than ever. We developed a real partnership in culinary imagination, and it is one of the most fruitful relationships I've ever had.

During this same time, Dr. Junger referred me to Dr. Habib Sadeghi, a doctor who has changed (and continues to change) my life. Dr. Sadeghi is a conventionally trained physician who also practices other integrative healing methods. He has immersed himself in the study of nutrition and osteopathic manipulative medicine, and uses techniques from the worlds of Ayurveda, Tibetan medicine, anthroposophical medicine, acupuncture, and energy healing. Basically, the kind of doctor I had been searching for. While I understood about the power of food and the power of detoxification, I had never really taken into account the emotional aspect of what we put into our bodies and why.

Dr. Sadeghi took my healing to another level. He asked what unspoken emotions could be contributing to my stress, and gave me another roster of tests, which revealed high levels of metals and a blood parasite, among other things—things that are often left undiagnosed and have incredibly negative impacts on our well-being. My whole family was tested for food sensitivities and allergies (something I would highly recommend to anyone looking to feel better, shed weight, etc.), and the results were enlightening. Everyone in my house is intolerant of gluten, dairy, and chickens' eggs, among many other surprising foods I had always thought were healthy. What do you feed kids who can't eat gluten when pasta and bread are their favorite things on earth? What do you give a kid for dessert who is allergic to cow's milk?

I decided that we needed to create this book, not only for my family, but also for anyone out there who struggles with finding truly delicious food to feed their family when health issues need to be addressed. So no matter if you are doing Dr. Junger's Clean Program, which focuses on the elimination diet; a lean-protein-based weight-loss diet; or a food allergy program that steers you away from gluten and dairy; or if you just want to focus a bit more on nutritious food—there are recipes and weekly menus here for you. And most importantly, no matter what you want or need to cut out, for whatever reason mealtimes should always feel happy. Not like a punishment. If I've learned anything, it's that it's all a process. "Falling off" your plan is part of it, not a reason to beat yourself up. It takes time to make these changes. It's all good. **—Gwyneth Paltrow**

How It All Got Really Good

Creating this book with Gwyneth changed my life. Learning to love and depend on the ingredients behind these recipes allowed me to transform not just my body, but also my relationship with food and with myself. Getting to know about healthy food and healthy living—for which I have to give quite a lot of credit to my dear blond friend—has simultaneously made me smaller and my world bigger.

For you to better understand the magnitude of this shift, I have to admit that I come from a long line of emotional eaters. In my family, food isn't just fuel—it's how we say "I love you." It's how we both reward and punish ourselves, how we connect, and even how we mourn. My mother's parents, who immigrated to America nearly a century ago, ran a bread bakery in Brooklyn. My father's grandfather built and ran a grain mill in Connecticut. White flour, in other words, runs in my blood.

While I was always a chubby kid, my weight never got out of control until I was a teenager. Even then, I was good at hiding it. I cultivated a wardrobe of comfortable, baggy button-down, men's shirts and a stack of dark (slimming!) jeans and masked deep-seated personal and physical insecurities with buckets of social and academic confidence. I played goalie and catcher so I wouldn't have to run but could still win the game. I was president of the student body, but skipped out on prom.

At the beginning of college I decided to get a handle on things. I started going to Weight Watchers, attending meetings at a local church with a group of women all about thirty years my senior. I started to pay attention to portion sizes and to confront emotional triggers, started to depend more on vegetables and stopped drinking soda. I thought I had it all figured out, so, naturally, I stopped going to meetings.

After college, I reached my highest weight ever. My relationship with food spiraled from relatively stable to completely out of hand. I wasn't paying attention to whether I was hungry or full. I wasn't aware that there was a distinction between what my body was craving and what my emotional state was craving. I remember watching weight-loss shows on television and realizing I weighed more than the contestants. I grew out of my favorite shirts and bought new ones and ripped out the tags that said what size they were. I felt disconnected from my body and stopped caring about how I treated it. It turned out that at my highest, I was at my lowest.

Dr. Habib Sadeghi, Gwyneth's doctor who generously penned our foreword, says that permanent weight loss is "a love issue—not a food issue." While I wish I had been able to read his book at that low moment in my life (he hadn't written it yet!), I decided then that my body wasn't an apartment I was renting, it was the house I would always live in. That turning point—that moment when something clicked—didn't occur because of a specific incident. I can't even pinpoint it to a specific hour or day or even month. It was a gradual change that had surprisingly little to do with my body and everything to do with an overall feeling of, in Dr. Sadeghi's words, self-love. It was all about understanding that changing my body would be a consequence of being a happier, more self-aware person and not the other way around.

For me, a quick fix wasn't an option. I didn't want a speedy, adrenaline-fueled weight loss without any deeper emotional change. I didn't want a Band-Aid. I wanted to work toward a healthier, more loving relationship with food. I wanted to respect food, since it's been the driving force throughout my entire life, the thing that informs my career and all my favorite moments. I didn't want to live resenting the thing I am constantly thinking about and working with.

So to say good-bye to sixty pounds (and counting!)—a consequence of bettering my relationship with both food and myself—I had to work slowly. I had to quite literally take small steps, had to work my way up from walking a block to running a couple of miles. I had to dig quite deep, had to separate my own weight issues from the ones I inherited, had to resolve old misunderstandings with people I loved, had to start believing in myself as much as everyone around me seemed to believe in me. I had to learn not to deflect compliments and to welcome help. I had to be nicer to myself. I had to let my hair down. I had to be open to spontaneity, had to trust my instincts and own my decisions. I had to let go. I had to change the way I cook and eat, had to find elegance through restraint, find tremendous beauty in simplicity, learn about new ingredients, and fall in love with them.

The recipes in this book are directly informed by this nourishing, positive relationship with food—a relationship that Gwyneth has helped me to nurture. We have cooked and enjoyed hundreds of meals together over the years, and this collection, created with so much love, presents the food we both believe most strongly in. These recipes, first and foremost, pay attention to the emotional power of food—and also happen to be amazingly good for you. They satisfy our nearly embarrassing, totally nerdy love of great cooking, and they also take care of our bodies. They hit nostalgic chords. They are how we regularly cook and are full of ingredients we swear by. They are full of memories, too: making this book with Gwyneth, who loves food like nobody else I know, wasn't just physically and emotionally transformative, it was also terrific fun. There is crazy joy in these pages.—**Julia Turshen**

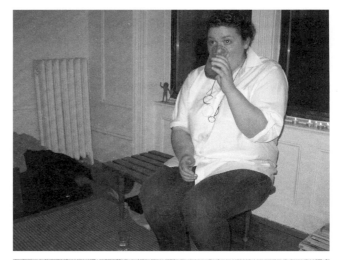

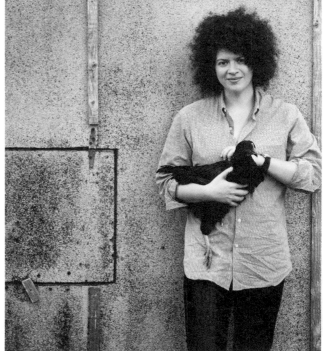

Top, Julia before; *bottom*, Julia now

Behind the Icons: How to Use This Book

No matter which plan you might be following—maybe you're eating according to your blood type, maybe you're on the Zone Diet or the Paleo diet or you're macrobiotic or you're following Dr. Junger's twenty-one-day Clean Program, or maybe you're following no plan at all and are looking for some guidance—the recipes in this book will take care of you. We've done our homework and learned about all of these diets, detox plans, and cleanses and have tried a lot of them, too. We've found that nearly all have the same tenets: eat whole foods, especially vegetables and lean protein and grains. Avoid white flour, sugar, and excess amounts of dairy. Cut out caffeine and booze if you consume too much of them.

There is no sugar in any recipe in this book. There is barely a trace of gluten and the recipes that make reference to it also offer gluten-free variations that are just as good. Other than a small handful of recipes that call for goat's milk or sheep's milk yogurt, a very digestible and probiotic-filled form of dairy, there is no dairy in this book. That's right—no butter, cheese, or cream. Not a single recipe calls for anything overly processed. This book is full of real, wholesome food—recipes that will make you feel lighter and full of energy, not weighed down. But it's all insanely delicious—comfort food that happens to follow the same protocols as all healthy eating plans.

If you're looking for more specificity from the recipes, we've included the following icons to help you navigate which recipes are suitable for different situations.

E Elimination Diet
V Vegan
P Protein-Packed

Before following any plan or diet, consult your doctor to find out what's best for you. We also highly recommend getting tested for food allergies, intolerances, and sensitivities. You'd be surprised by how many undesirable things we're exposed to in our food supply—arsenic has been found in rice, mold in grains—not to mention the heavy metals and other toxic substances we encounter on a daily basis in our environments. The good news is that awareness of all of this, coupled with a good diet, can both heal and prevent all sorts of issues. Talk to your doctor about tests for food allergies and sensitivities—the more you know about your body, the more easily you can help yourself feel great.

A note to UK readers

Measurements
The recipes use American cups (as well as imperial measurements) so you'll need a set of these to prepare the dishes. Measuring cups are now widely available and are very easy to use. They measure by volume: on page 303 there's a short conversion chart you may find useful if you prefer to measure your liquid using a metric measuring jug. To measure solid ingredients using cups simply scoop, pour, or pack according to the ingredient—it's a bit like using big tablespoons. Cups are very convenient for things like flour and nuts and although using them for ingredients such as vegetables and herbs may seem a little unfamiliar, remember this is all good stuff so throwing in a little bit more or less isn't going to be a problem.

Ingredients
This book is all about the good stuff—healthy, natural ingredients that you can find in good grocers, markets, and health food stores, so the vast majority of ingredients should be familiar to you and readily available. However, there are a few that are a little more unusual outside the US. These are mostly ingredients for Mexican-influenced dishes—plus a few flavorings and Asian ingredients—but these are available in good delis or online retailers: try coolchile.co.uk for Mexican ingredients, japancentre.com for Asian ingredients, and panzers.co.uk for hard-to-find American foods such as Old Bay seasoning. And, of course, you can substitute a similar ingredient or flavor if that's more convenient. I'm sure that you are aware of many of the names we have in the US for common ingredients, but here are the ones we use a lot in these recipes: arugula is rocket, scallions are spring onions, cilantro is coriander, navy beans are haricot beans, beets are beetroot, Napa cabbage is Chinese leaf, and baking soda is bicarbonate of soda.

Oven temperatures
The oven temperatures used in the recipes are in degrees Fahrenheit, which is commonly used for ovens in US. On page 303 you'll find a chart giving the degrees Celsius and gas mark equivalents.

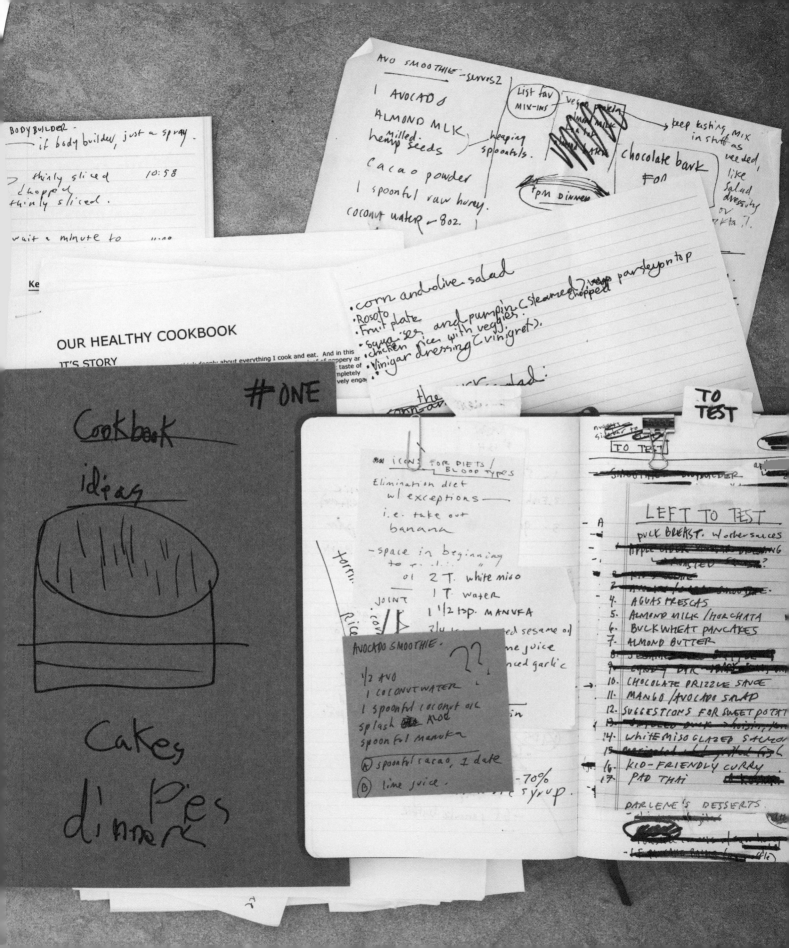

Pantry

Julia here. Once, after a long day of work and travel, Gwyneth and I found ourselves late at night with a small group of hungry people in a kitchen that hadn't been used in months. We were more or less in the middle of nowhere and all the stores were closed. There was mustard in the fridge and a package of duck bacon in the freezer. Oil, vinegar, and some chickpea flour were in the cupboard. Like a prize, a perfectly ripe avocado emerged from Gwyneth's carry-on. Armed with a flashlight, I made a quick trip to the vegetable garden. It was June, so the greens had just shot up, and I gathered fistfuls of arugula, a bunch of chives, and some rosemary. We got to work. We put a cast-iron pan into the oven to get hot and mixed the chickpea flour with water, salt, and olive oil. We poured the batter into the hot pan, sprinkled the top with fresh rosemary, and put it back into the oven. While the duck bacon was cooking, Gwyneth whisked together a simple vinaigrette and packed it with chopped chives. I washed the greens and diced the avocado, and she coated both with the dressing and then crumbled in the salty, crispy duck bacon. We all stood at the counter and feasted on the salad and sliced ourselves wedges of the chickpea pancake/frittata/baked-polenta-ish concoction. Something from seemingly nothing, the meal was a testament to the power of a pantry, no matter how sparsely it's stocked. With only a handful of ingredients, a comforting, healthy meal with real substance can be achieved anywhere, anytime. All of the recipes in this book depend entirely on great ingredients. Whether you've got room for every spice and grain or space for just a few, keeping good staples around is the first step toward cooking well at home. In the following pages, you'll find the ingredients we depend on the most. When we had questions about certain pantry items, we asked Dr. Alejandro Junger to share his expertise. You'll find his thoughts in places marked "Alejandro says."

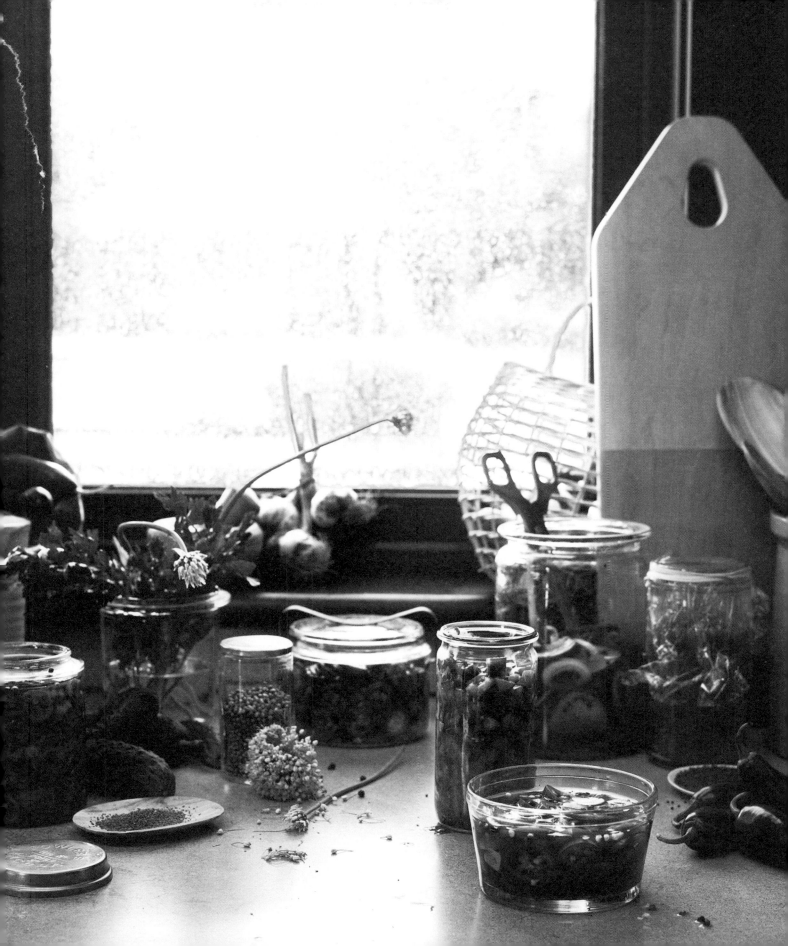

IN THE FRIDGE

Fresh Produce!

Berries, dark leafy greens, leeks and scallions, carrots and cucumbers, fresh chili peppers and ginger, plenty of fresh herbs, asparagus, and more…Our lives would be bland and our bodies weak without plenty of fresh produce.

Jars and Bottles

Vegenaise: We basically can't live without Vegenaise—it's a little out of control. We prefer it over regular mayonnaise, we schlep it if we're going somewhere they don't sell it, we spread it on just about everything (see Avocado Toast on page 34), we use it instead of oil in baked goods (see The Brownie Recipe That Could on page 252), we mix it into dressings (see Creamy Parsley Dressing on page 61 and Mexican Green Goddess on page 57), and we save the jars to store salad dressings and homemade pickles in.

Good-quality maple syrup: We use maple syrup way beyond pancakes and waffles (but don't get us wrong, we love it on them!). It's one of our favorite natural sweeteners and is full of antioxidants and zinc. It's said to be great for digestion and even muscle recovery, and we depend on it to sweeten dressings, sauces, and baked goods.

Mustard: Good-quality Dijon mustard and coarse seeded mustard find their way into lots of our dressings.

Pickles and kimchi: Whether it's a full-sour Bubbies pickle or a tangle of spicy cabbage kimchi, fermented foods add assertive punches of flavor to and alongside our dishes. It doesn't hurt that fermented vegetables are said to reduce cholesterol and support the digestive system and are a huge boost for the immune system, so much so that kimchi is considered a cancer-fighting food. Kimchi is available at your neighborhood Asian market, at Hmart .com, and at Whole Foods, and is increasingly found in major grocery stores.

Miso paste: Offering the same health benefits as pickles and kimchi, miso paste is made of fermented soybeans. Its flavor enlivens lots of our dressings and sauces (check out the Carrot-Ginger Dressing on page 65 and Lee's Hoisin Sauce on page 275). We mostly use sweet white miso and red miso made from soybeans, but misos made with brown rice and barley are really nice, too. Experiment to find which ones you like best, since they keep in the fridge forever!

A Note on Miso: *Why is miso good for you?*

Alejandro says…
    "Miso is a fermented food and therefore has great benefits for health, such as a high content of readily absorbable B vitamins, pre- and probiotics, and minerals. Always go for GMO-free miso (that's miso without any genetically modified organisms); organic is preferable."

Raw coconut water: Basically nature's sports drink, raw coconut water has more potassium per serving than a banana and is full of electrolytes. While it's pretty perfect on its own, especially during or after a workout, we also like to use it in smoothies and even in some recipes like Black Rice with Fresh Coconut (see page 183). If you have access to fresh, young coconut and are fearless with a knife, that's the way to go. If you'd prefer something a bit more convenient and less messy, our favorite brand of coconut water, by far, is Harmless Harvest, which is sold at Whole Foods.

Almond milk: Nearly all of our shakes and smoothies would suffer without our favorite cow's milk alternative. We use almond milk in lots of baked goods, too. When we have time, we love to make our own (see page 220), but there's no shame in buying it—always look for plain unsweetened almond milk (unless you're making Bernardo's Pumpkin Pie Shake, on page 209, which calls for unsweetened vanilla almond milk).

Dairy

We have mostly stayed away from dairy in this book (though if you put a ripe, runny, stinky cheese in front of either of us…watch out), but occasionally you'll see recipes that call for plain, full-fat sheep's or goat's milk yogurt (which we've been able to find at Whole Foods and health food stores all across the country). Way more digestible and less allergenic than cow's milk varieties, yogurt made from sheep's and goat's milk is full of protein, healthy bacteria, and probiotics. If you can find raw versions of either yogurt, so much the better. If needed or desired, regular cow's milk yogurt can be substituted.

Proteins

Eggs: We use only organic eggs, preferably local ones from chickens, ducks, and even quails.

Fish: Wherever we are, we look for fish that's been caught as close to our kitchen as possible. We tend to lean toward wild salmon and fillets of small white fish, things like flounder, fluke, and sole. You'll also see striped bass called for in a lot of the fish recipes—that's because it swims in the waters close to Gwyneth's summer home, where we do a lot of cooking. Feel free to substitute whatever is best near you, and become friends with your fishmonger—he or she will point you toward whatever is freshest.

A Note on Shellfish: *Why no shellfish when you're trying to eat cleanly?*

Alejandro says…

"Shellfish are included in my list of foods to avoid, but mostly for the twenty-one-day duration of the Clean Program. I suggest this for two reasons. They are often the cause of food allergies and sensitivities, plus there are reports that they contain mercury. Mercury levels are much lower in shellfish than in large fish, such as tuna. If one is tested for mercury body burden and it is found not to be elevated, shellfish consumption is fine. Shellfish contain good lean protein and beneficial nonsaturated fats, as well as iodine, essential for thyroid hormone production and an optimal metabolism."

Poultry: Organic chicken, turkey, and duck find themselves in our refrigerators in all forms—whole birds, ground meat, fresh sausages, even bacon.

Red meat: Gwyneth eats zero red meat and Julia eats a tiny bit here and there, but we both often make it for other people in our lives (mostly men…).

A Note on Soy and Tofu: *What are your thoughts on soy, specifically tofu? Is eating it in moderation okay?*

Alejandro says…

"Not all soy products are created equal, starting with the soybeans themselves, which could be from GMOs. GMOs are plants whose genes have been tampered with, and there is more and more evidence that this practice poses potential threats to human health. One example of what is done to genetically modified plants is the introduction into the cell's nucleus of genes that make the plant itself into a pesticide. When insects eat this kind of GMO, they die. Common sense tells me this cannot be good for humans to consume, either.

"The addition of preservatives, coloring agents, smelling agents, texturizing agents, and other chemicals can turn any product into a slow-acting poison, soy or not, so make sure you choose products that are naturally prepared and free of these chemicals.

"Another problem with soy and its derivative products is the presence of phytoestrogens (*phyto* = plant). These molecules can mimic the effects of estrogen in the body by binding to estrogen receptors, and the consequence can be the disruption of hormonal balance. One of the common ways I see this is as the inability to get pregnant. I have known many women to get pregnant soon after stopping all soy products. Soy isoflavones are thought to compete with iodine at the thyroid level, and some studies show decreased thyroid activity, which corrected after soy was discontinued. This is an important fact to consider in choosing soy products for your kids in the first years of life, when a decrease in thyroid activity can impair normal growth and development. I personally avoid most soy products for my kids and do not recommend soy-based formulas for babies.

"But soy isoflavones also have some positive effects, such as reducing the incidence of hormone-dependent cancers, and soy can help menopausal women relieve symptoms, such as hot flashes, typical of this phase of life.

"Another beneficial aspect of soy is the high content of ALA (alpha-linolenic acid) in its oils, which may in part be what makes the Japanese people a population with one of the lowest rates of coronary artery disease. Together with soy's high fiber content, that high ALA content can keep your heart from getting sick.

"All this can be somewhat confusing, so to boil it down I would say this: Use soy products in moderation and check the ingredients to make sure each product is not from GMO soy and does not contain toxic chemicals."

IN THE FREEZER

Gluten-free bread: We like Food For Life's millet bread and rice bread, or, for days with a little bit of gluten, Ezekiel 4:9 sprouted grain bread. Keep a loaf in your freezer for toast and sandwiches.

Peas: We reach for frozen peas all the time, especially to add a bit of brightness to rice dishes like Risotto with Peas + Greens (see page 180), Chicken + Turkey Sausage Paella (see page 184), and Mexican Tomato Rice (see page 183).

IN THE SPICE CABINET

Maldon sea salt: This is always in close reach—it's the best salt in the world, as far as we're concerned.

Freshly ground black pepper: It makes a huge difference to use a peppermill instead of preground pepper.

Dried red chili: We use pinches of traditional red chili flakes (like the ones you see at pizzerias) in tons of stuff, especially in a hot skillet with garlic and olive oil before dark greens like broccoli rabe (see Broccoli Rabe with Garlic + Red Chili, page 154) hit the pan. Gochugaru, coarse Korean red chili flakes, are also great to have on hand to sprinkle on things like Grilled Corn, Korean Style (see page 158) and Avocado Toast (see page 34). They're available at lots of Asian grocery stores, or check out Hmart.com.

Pimentón: This smoked paprika from Spain is one of our favorite ingredients, since it easily offers serious flavor that makes things taste as if you've been slow-cooking for hours. It comes in sweet (*dulce*) and hot (*picante*). We like both, but you can always use sweet if you like things a bit more mild, and hot if you like more kick.

Chinese five-spice powder: A blend of ground ginger, cloves, black pepper, cinnamon, and fennel (the mixture varies a bit), Chinese five-spice powder is a beautiful combination that we love to incorporate into lots of dishes, especially ones with sweet potatoes (see Sweet Potato + Five-Spice Muffins on page 41 and A Plain Roasted Sweet Potato on page 152).

Old Bay seasoning: Made primarily of celery seed and paprika, Old Bay is one of our most beloved flavor combinations, especially for anything involving crispy fish (see Best Gluten-Free Fish Fingers on page 234).

Vege-Sal: An old-school seasoning blend made of salt and ground dehydrated vegetables, Vege-Sal is like a hippie's Mrs. Dash and we heart it, especially on Avocado Toast (see page 34) or on A Hard-Boiled Egg (see page 278).

ON THE COUNTER

Fresh produce: Lemons, limes, garlic, shallots, onions, sweet potatoes, apples, and avocados...we can't get enough.

A Note on Nightshades: *What's wrong with nightshades?*

Alejandro says...

"There is nothing wrong with nightshades; in fact, they have amazing properties and health benefits. The only reason I exclude them in the elimination diet during the Clean Program is because some people may be sensitive to solanine, an alkaloid present in nightshades that can turn on the inflammatory process, especially around the joints. Once the twenty-one-day detox is complete, I encourage people to reintroduce nightshades in the right manner (following the reintroduction phase correctly) and determine whether they are sensitive to solanine or not. Some people are sensitive and would benefit from limiting their consumption, or stopping it altogether, but most people are not, and they would actually benefit from consuming these amazing vegetables."

IN THE CUPBOARD

For Baking

All-purpose gluten-free flour: We are really into Cup4Cup, a blend made by Thomas Keller that's sold at Williams-Sonoma. It's the gluten-free blend that they use at his famous restaurant the French Laundry, and you can substitute it cup for cup (hence the name) for regular all-purpose flour. We also recommend Bob's Red Mill All-Purpose Baking Flour, which you can easily get on the Bob's Red Mill website or at Whole Foods and most health food stores. In England, Doves Farm makes amazing flours, and their gluten-free bread flour is a dream. Whichever brand you choose, check to see if xanthan gum (a binder that helps give gluten-free baked goods structure) is included. If it's not, we find that adding ½ teaspoon of xanthan gum for every cup of all-purpose gluten-free flour works perfectly.

Almond meal: Simply made of ground almonds, almond meal is an amazing flour substitute, and we especially love it as part of a crunchy topping in Flourless Anything Crumble (see page 259). Bob's Red Mill makes a great one. Or you can make your own by grinding blanched almonds in a powerful blender.

Quinoa flakes: Quinoa flakes are a terrific gluten-free, protein-packed substitute for oats.

Sweet Stuff

Xylitol: Xylitol is a natural sweetener made from fruit and vegetable fibers. We know it sounds super-medical and scientific, but it's actually an incredibly healthy alternative to sugar, is remarkably good for your teeth, and works really well in baking.

A Note on Xylitol: *What are your thoughts on xylitol?*

Alejandro says...

"Xylitol tastes much better than many other nonsugar sweeteners. It looks like sugar, it feels like sugar, and it mixes with other ingredients easily, like sugar, without sugar's high glycemic index. Occasionally it can cause upset stomach. People should try it and see how it works for them individually."

Manuka honey: Said to be healing and full of antibacterial and antiviral properties, manuka honey is a bona fide superfood. It comes from honeybees that feast on manuka bushes in New Zealand. From a culinary perspective, it's got a strong flavor, so we use it sparingly. We buy it at Whole Foods and our local health food stores. You can also get it online.

Fish sauce: Made of fermented fish, fish sauce is our pungent, salty secret ingredient in many recipes that have southeast Asian influences. If you've never used fish sauce before, don't be put off by its distinctly assertive smell—a little goes a long way, and its flavor is irreplaceable.

A Note on Fish Sauce: *Is fish sauce allowed on the elimination diet?*

Alejandro says…
    "Not all fish sauce is created equal. In essence, if it is free of toxic chemicals, fish sauce should be fine. But many of the fish sauces available are very processed and full of chemicals; some may even include MSG. Make sure to read the ingredients carefully before using any packaged fish sauce."

Vinegars: We reach for vinegar all the time, especially when making dressings. White wine, red wine, sherry, apple cider, brown rice, and regular rice vinegar make the most appearances in our kitchens.

Soy sauce: Made of fermented soybeans, soy sauce helps just about anything taste better. Most soy sauces have wheat in them, so if you have a gluten sensitivity, be sure to look for naturally fermented, gluten-free varieties (which are readily available).

Bragg Liquid Aminos: A salty, gluten-free liquid protein concentrate. We use Bragg's anywhere you would use soy sauce (it's also made from soybeans).

Toasted sesame oil and hot toasted sesame oil: We love the robust, nutty flavor of toasted sesame oil—both the regular kind and the spicy variety, which has red chili in it.

Almond butter: Spread on toast, a brown rice cake, or an apple, almond butter is a great snack. But it's also a wonderful ingredient, especially in shakes like the Almond + Kale Smoothie on page 207 and in sauces like the Miso-Almond Sauce on page 162.

Canned tomatoes: The base of Go-To Tomato Sauce (see page 273), Chicken + White Bean Chili (see page 102), and Turkey + Black Bean Chili with Sweet Potatoes (see page 106). We love using canned tomatoes, since they're peeled and ready to go and also have great flavor.

Dried mushrooms: When rehydrated with boiling water, dried mushrooms make a quick, delicious vegan broth with great depth of flavor (check out Many-Mushroom Soup on page 81 and Polenta with Shiitakes + Fried Leeks on page 188).

A Few Tools We Can't Live Without

Microplane graters: We rely on these super-sharp graters, especially for pureeing ginger and garlic and zesting lemons and limes.

Vitamix blender: Worth the investment—the most powerful blender on the market, the Vitamix is responsible for our creamy shakes and smoothies and dressings and our rich, luxurious soups without any cream. When we say "powerful blender," this is what we're referring to.

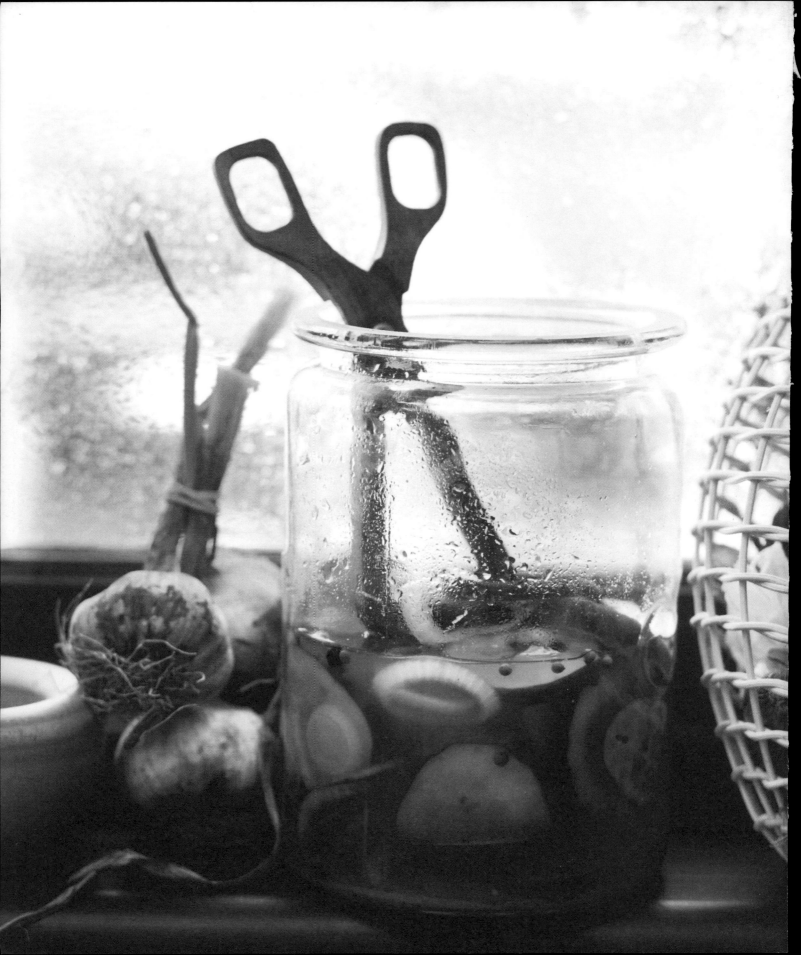

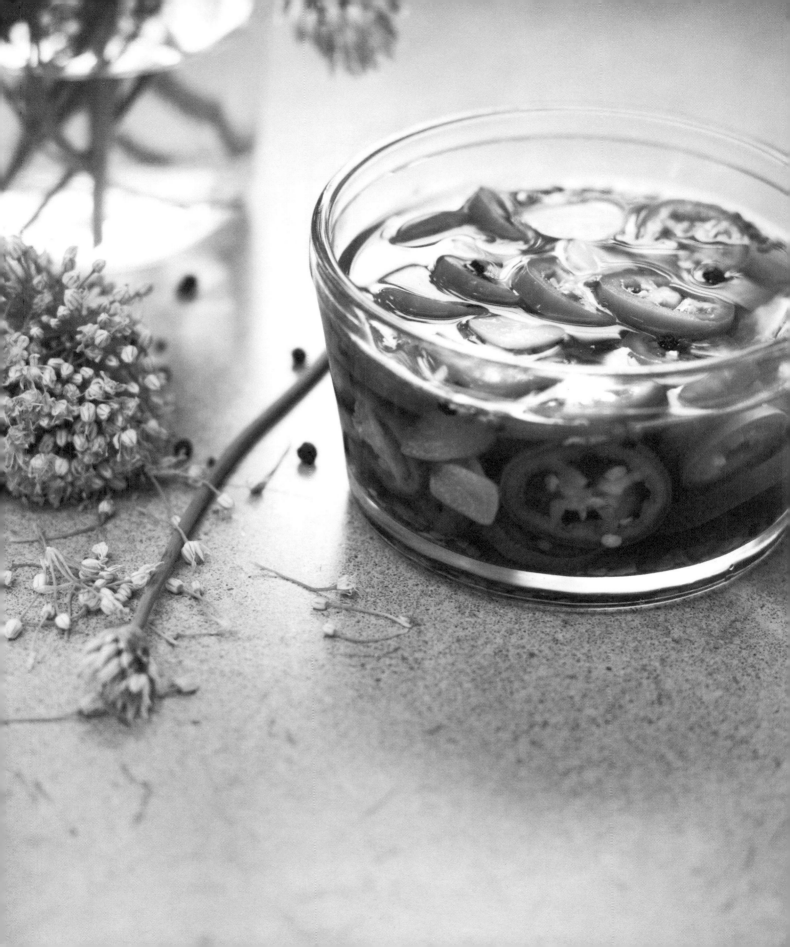

MORNING TIME

A toasted bagel, a pile of pancakes, a stack of toast, not to mention the muffins, scones, and generous pours of cheap cereal that tempt us all—morning-time food can often veer toward empty-carb, gluten-filled butter city. But even without wheat, dairy, or sugar, we've managed to keep nostalgia and comfort in mind throughout this chapter—you'll find "buttermilk" waffles, banana muffins, delicious granola, and more. The following recipes are my favorite healthy ways to start the day and get off on the right foot.

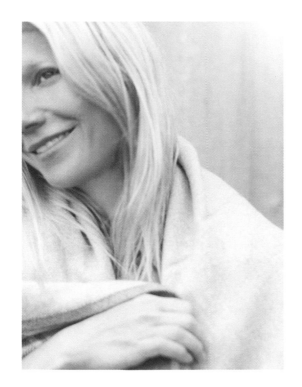
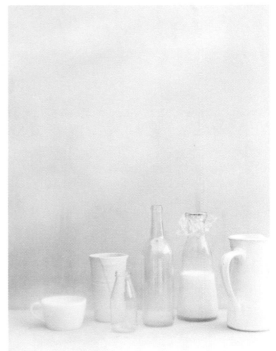

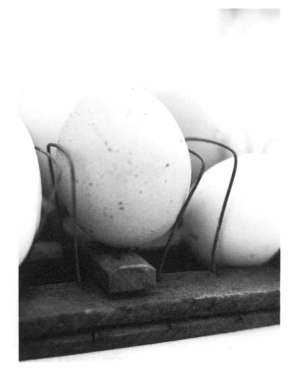

QUINOA GRANOLA WITH OLIVE OIL + MAPLE SYRUP

I'm allergic to oats, so this morning granola (which can also be eaten by the handful as an afternoon snack) is a healthy way to begin my day. Serve with a bit of fresh fruit and goat's milk yogurt or almond milk if you like.

Makes 6 cups

V Vegan **P** Protein-Packed

½ cup extra virgin olive oil
½ cup good-quality maple syrup
3 cups quinoa flakes
Coarse sea salt
1¼ cups roughly chopped raw walnuts
1¼ cups roughly chopped raw pumpkin seeds
¾ cup roughly chopped dried figs (stems
    discarded)
¾ cup roughly chopped pitted prunes

Preheat the oven to 400°F.

Whisk together the olive oil and maple syrup in a large mixing bowl and add the quinoa flakes, stirring to combine thoroughly. Evenly spread the quinoa on a parchment-lined baking sheet and sprinkle with a pinch of salt. Roast, stirring now and then, until the flakes are dried and crunchy and a lovely golden brown, about 25 minutes. Let the quinoa mixture cool completely before mixing with the remaining ingredients. Store in a glass jar for up to 2 weeks.

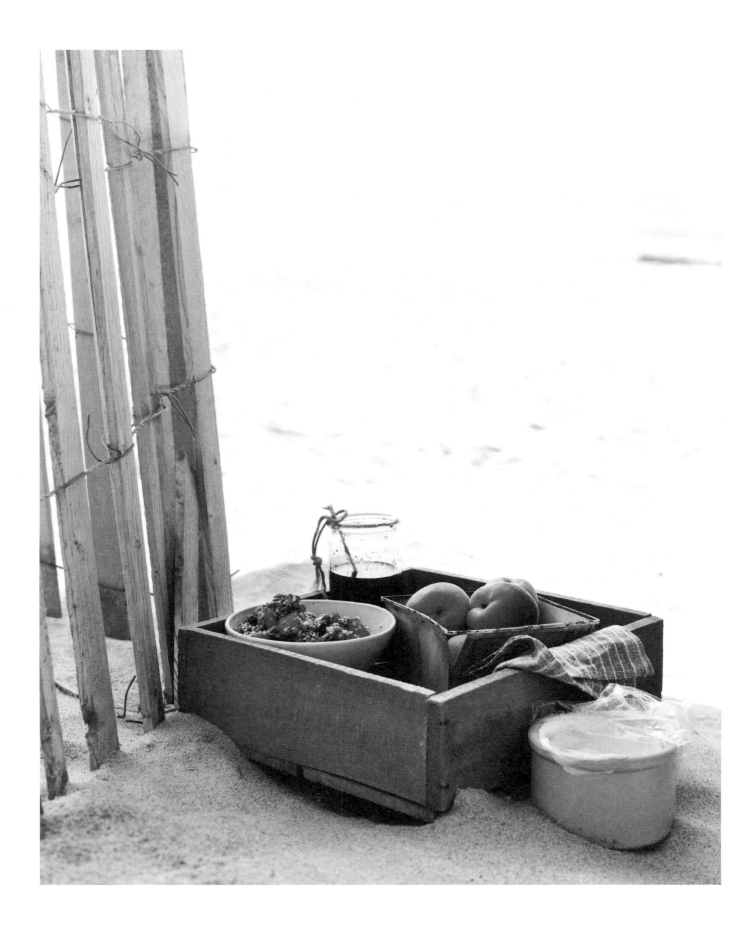

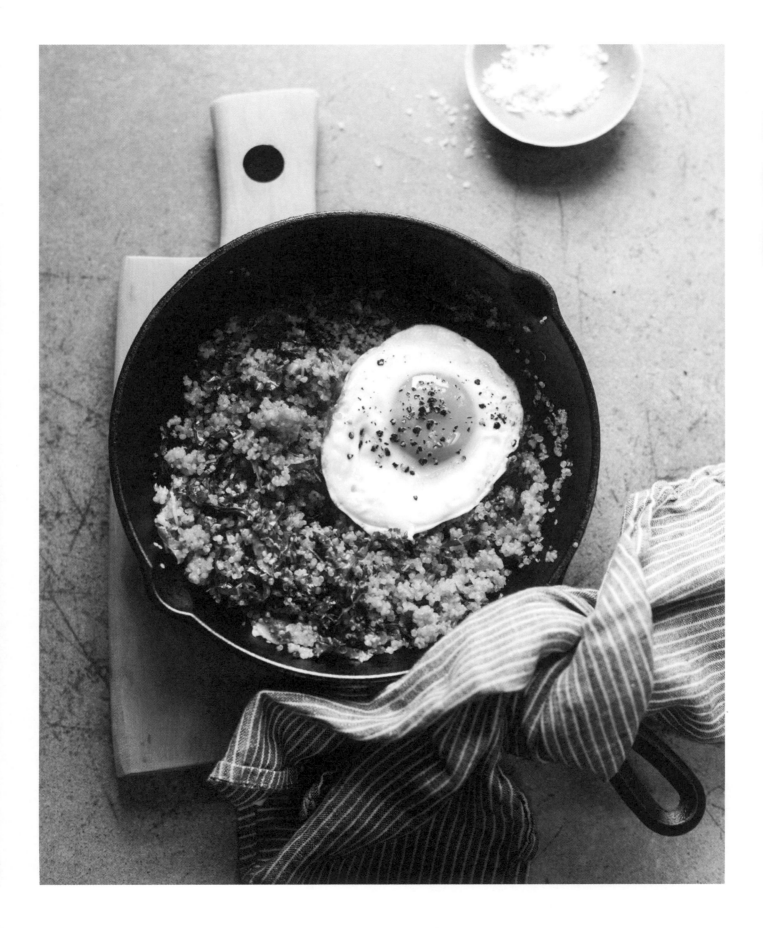

LEFTOVER QUINOA, TWO WAYS

Cooked quinoa is a great, useful staple to have on hand at all times, especially in the morning.

QUITE SAVORY

Serves 1

P Protein-Packed

2 tablespoons extra virgin olive oil
1 garlic clove, finely minced
2 large leaves of kale (stems discarded), finely
       shredded
½ cup Perfectly Cooked Quinoa (see page 178)
Coarse sea salt
Freshly ground black pepper
A Poached Egg (see page 278) or An Olive
       Oil–Fried Egg (see page 278)
1 scallion, white and light green parts only, very
       finely sliced

Heat the oil and garlic over medium heat in a small skillet until the garlic begins to soften, just 1 minute. Add the shredded kale and cook, stirring now and then, until the kale is wilted, 2 to 3 minutes. Add the quinoa and cook, stirring, until warmed through, another 2 minutes. Season the mixture to taste with salt and pepper. Place the mixture in a shallow bowl or on a plate, top with the egg, and sprinkle with the scallions. Add a final grind of black pepper if you like.

A BIT SWEET

Serves 1

E Elimination Diet **V** Vegan **P** Protein-Packed

¾ cup Perfectly Cooked Quinoa (see page 178)
½ cup unsweetened almond milk
Toppings: sliced toasted almonds, a drizzle
       of maple syrup, a chopped date, sliced
       banana, chopped dried figs, toasted
       walnuts, fresh blueberries, unsweetened
       shredded coconut, etc.

Combine the quinoa and almond milk in a small saucepan set over medium heat and cook, stirring, until warmed through, just 2 or 3 minutes. Transfer the mixture to a bowl and add whatever combination of toppings you like.

POWER OATMEAL

This oatmeal elevates the usual morning porridge into a breakfast loaded not only with layers of flavor and texture, but also with magnesium from the buckwheat, omega-3 fatty acids from the flaxseeds, and, from the sesame seeds, surprising amounts of copper (a vital element that's especially good for you if you suffer from arthritis).

Serves 4

V Vegan

½ cup old-fashioned rolled oats
½ cup buckwheat
1½ cups unsweetened almond milk
1½ cups water
Pinch of sea salt
¼ cup ground flaxseeds
1 tablespoon toasted sesame seeds

Combine the oats, buckwheat, almond milk, water, and salt in a heavy saucepan set over high heat. Bring to a boil, then turn the heat to low. Simmer the oatmeal uncovered, stirring now and then, until very soft, 20 to 25 minutes. Stir in the flaxseeds and sesame seeds and serve.

AVOCADO TOAST

V Vegan

Truthfully, this is the one "recipe" both Julia and I make and eat most often! And it's not even a recipe. Toast a piece of your favorite healthy, preferably gluten-free bread. Spread it generously with Vegenaise and top with a few slices of perfectly ripe avocado, ever so gently pressing the avocado into the bread. Hit it with a nice pinch of Maldon salt or Vege-Sal and a few grinds of black pepper. That's it. Sometimes we squeeze a tiny bit of lemon over it or add some zip with fruity red chili flakes (like Aleppo pepper or gochugaru, coarse Korean red chili flakes), but really it's the holy trinity of Vegenaise, avocado, and salt that makes this like a favorite pair of jeans—so reliable and easy and always just what you want.

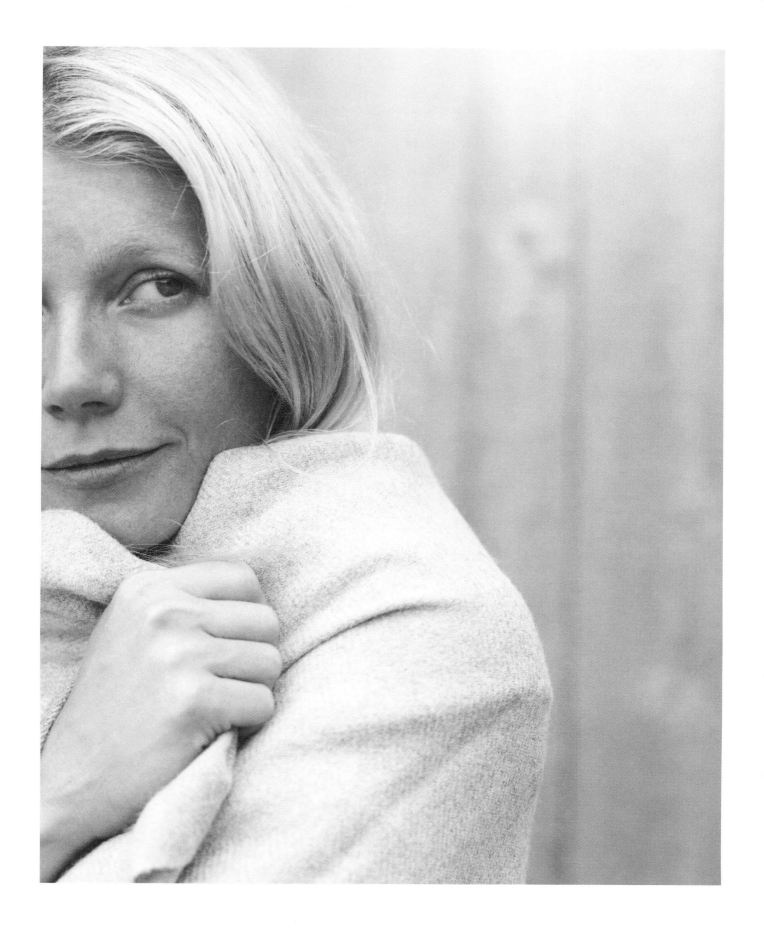

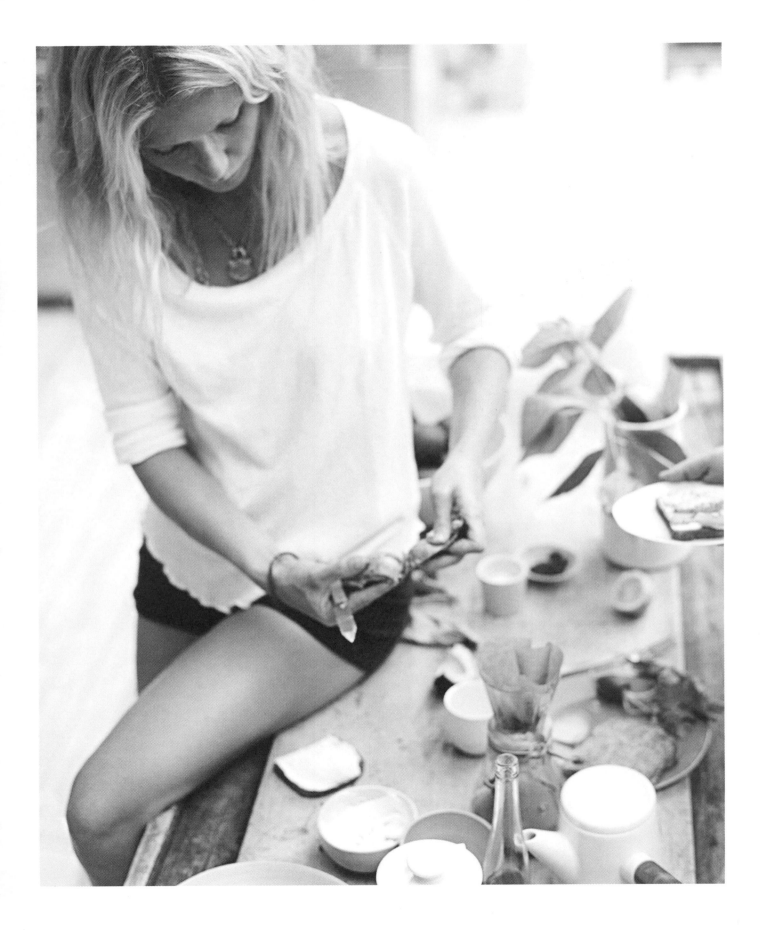

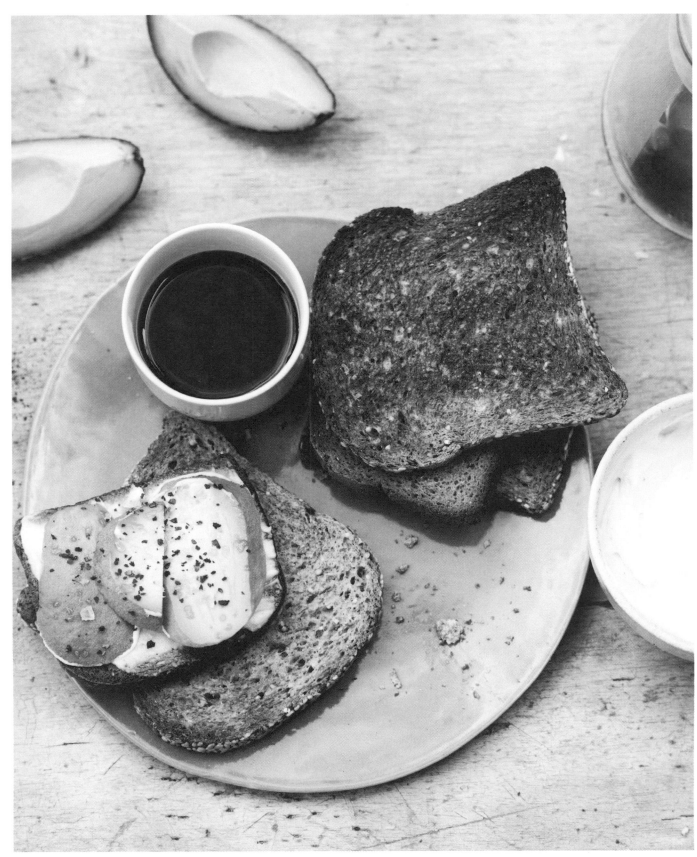

Avocado Toast (page 34)

POACHED EGGS WITH GARLICKY SPINACH + CRISPY TURKEY BACON

Serves any number; we like 2 eggs, 2 strips of bacon, and a pile of spinach for each person

Ⓟ Protein-Packed

Another nonrecipe breakfast deal, but I love this combination so much I couldn't leave it out. This makes for a lot of pans to wash, but on a Saturday or Sunday morning it's really worth it. For each serving, simply sauté a sliced garlic clove in a glug (about 2 tablespoons) of olive oil, add a few big handfuls of baby spinach, stir to combine, and watch the spinach wilt till it's barely there. Season to taste with salt and serve alongside two poached eggs (See A Poached Egg, page 278) and a few strips of crispy turkey bacon. The moment you get a taste of egg yolk with the garlic and greens and that salty, smoky bite of bacon…yes, please.

"BUTTERMILK" WAFFLES

These gluten-, dairy-, and sugar-free waffles provide a homey, comforting breakfast. You won't know what you're missing. This batter makes great pancakes, too—simply add an extra ½ cup soy milk and cook them as you would any other pancake.

Serves 4 (makes 8 waffles)

Ⓥ Vegan

3 cups soy milk
2 tablespoons freshly squeezed lemon juice
2 teaspoons pure vanilla extract
2 tablespoons good-quality maple syrup, plus more for serving
1 cup all-purpose gluten-free flour (if the flour doesn't include xanthan gum, add ½ teaspoon)
1 cup brown rice flour
1½ teaspoons baking powder
A large pinch of sea salt
Canola or grapeseed oil cooking spray for your waffle maker

Mix the soy milk and lemon juice in a bowl and let them sit for 10 minutes, or until the mixture begins to thicken and curdle. Whisk in the vanilla and maple syrup. In another mixing bowl, whisk together the flours, baking powder, and salt. Combine the wet and dry ingredients, being careful not to overmix.

Heat your waffle maker according to the manufacturer's instructions. Grease with a little oil and cook your waffles until they're nicely browned on both sides, 4 to 7 minutes, depending on your machine. Serve with maple syrup.

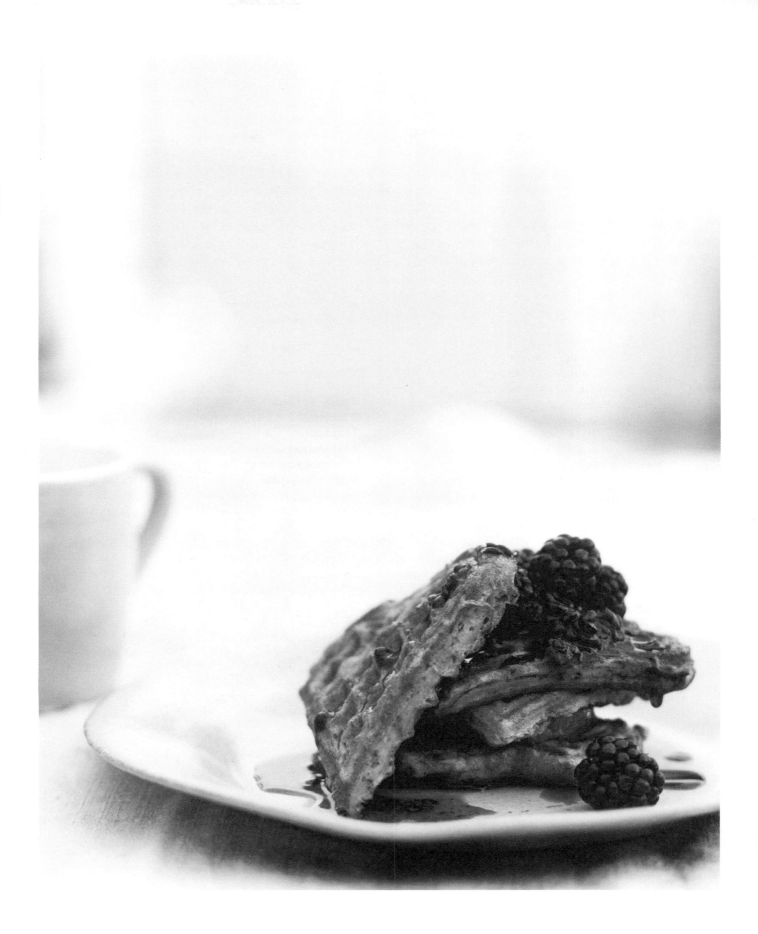

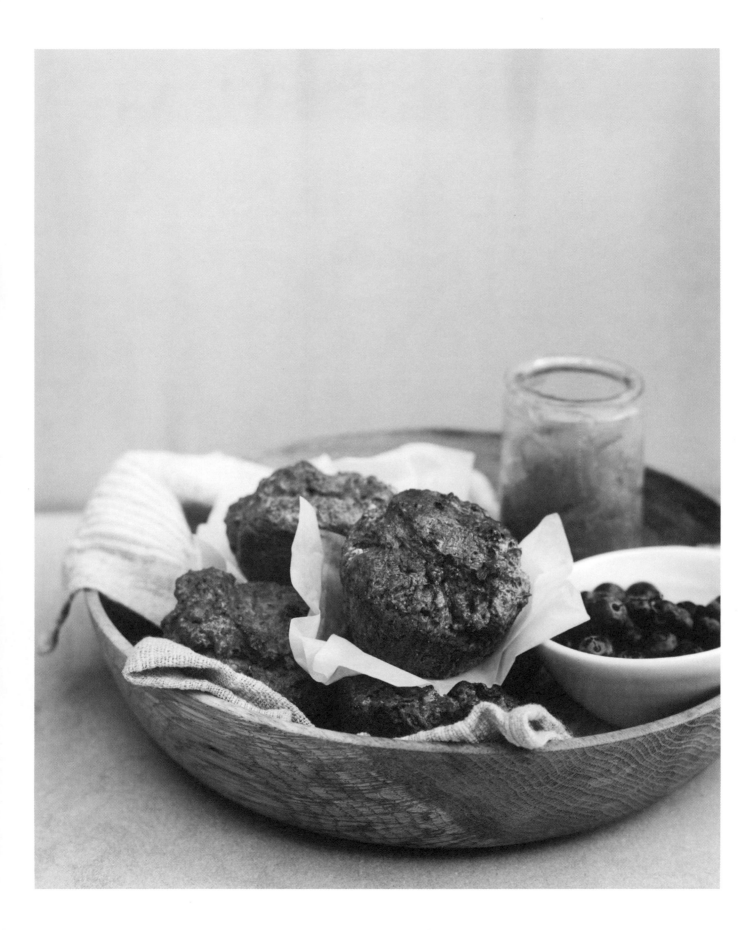

SWEET POTATO + FIVE-SPICE MUFFINS

Gluten-free baking is not for the faint of heart. At first as we tested this recipe, we produced heavy or bizarrely textured muffins, but we finally hit the nail on the head with the perfect mix of ingredients. These muffins are super-tasty and are always a smashing success in my house.

Makes a dozen muffins

Ⓥ Vegan

1 large sweet potato
½ cup extra virgin olive oil
½ cup unsweetened almond milk
¾ cup good-quality maple syrup or xylitol,
    plus 2 extra tablespoons for brushing
    the muffins
1 teaspoon pure vanilla extract
2 cups gluten-free flour (if the flour doesn't
    include xanthan gum, add 1 teaspoon)
2 teaspoons baking powder
2 teaspoons baking soda
1½ tablespoons Chinese five-spice powder
½ teaspoon fine sea salt

Preheat the oven to 400°F. Prick the sweet potato a few times with a paring knife or a fork. Bake until soft (when a paring knife can cut through with zero resistance), about 1 hour. Set the sweet potato aside until it's completely cool.

Peel the sweet potato, discard the skin, and mash the flesh in a mixing bowl with a fork. Whisk the olive oil, almond milk, maple syrup or xylitol, and vanilla into the sweet potato. In a separate bowl, whisk together the flour, baking powder, baking soda, five-spice powder, and salt. Fold the dry ingredients into the wet ingredients.

Line a 12-cup muffin tin with paper liners and evenly distribute the muffin batter among the cups.

Bake for 20 to 25 minutes, or until a toothpick comes out clean, brushing the tops with the extra maple syrup during the last 5 minutes of baking. Let the muffins cool before serving.

BUCKWHEAT + BANANA PANCAKES

This combination of nutty buckwheat and sweet, sticky banana is just great. You could sprinkle chopped walnuts on the pancakes as they're cooking for a full-on pancake-meets-banana-bread experience. These happen to be vegan, but they don't taste like it. Buckwheat flour adds a lot of value to these pancakes–it's rich in nutrients like calcium, iron, B vitamins, and protein, and it's gluten free.

Serves 4 (makes a dozen 4-inch pancakes)

Ⓥ Vegan

1¼ cups soy milk or rice milk
1 tablespoon freshly squeezed lemon juice
1 tablespoon vegetable oil
1 tablespoon good-quality maple syrup, plus
    more for serving
½ cup buckwheat flour
½ cup white spelt flour, if you can tolerate a bit
    of gluten, or ½ cup all-purpose gluten-free
    flour if you can't
1 teaspoon baking soda
½ teaspoon sea salt
Coconut oil or any neutral oil (like canola,
    grapeseed, or safflower oil) for cooking
2 bananas, thinly sliced

Whisk together the soy milk or rice milk, lemon juice, vegetable oil, and maple syrup in a small bowl. In a slightly larger bowl, whisk together the flours, baking soda, and salt. Add the wet ingredients to the dry ingredients and stir until just combined.

Heat a large nonstick skillet or griddle over medium-high heat. Slick it with a bit of oil and ladle in as many pancakes as can fit comfortably. Place a few slices of banana on top of each pancake. Cook for about 1½ minutes on the first side, or until the surface is covered with small bubbles and the underside is nicely browned. Flip and cook for about 1 minute on the second side. Repeat the process until you run out of batter. Serve stacked high, with plenty of maple syrup.

MILLET-FIG MUFFINS

Not too sweet, these muffins are full of wholesome ingredients, including millet, which adds great texture, and flaxseeds, which provide a full hit of fiber. Brought together with savory olive oil, these make not just a great breakfast but a great after-school or postworkout snack.

Makes a dozen muffins

Ⓥ Vegan

2 cups gluten-free flour (if the flour doesn't
    include xanthan gum, add 1 teaspoon)
½ cup raw millet
2 teaspoons baking powder
2 teaspoons baking soda
A big pinch of fine sea salt
1 teaspoon ground ginger
⅓ cup ground flaxseeds
⅔ cup good-quality maple syrup
⅔ cup unsweetened almond milk
⅔ cup extra virgin olive oil
1 cup chopped dried figs

Preheat the oven to 400°F and line a 12-cup muffin tin with paper liners.

Whisk the flour, millet, baking powder, baking soda, salt, ginger, and flaxseeds together in a large bowl. In another bowl whisk together the maple syrup, almond milk, and olive oil. Toss the chopped figs in a small bowl with a spoonful of the dry ingredients (this keeps the figs from sinking to the bottom of the muffins). Fold the wet ingredients into the dry ingredients until just combined, then fold in the figs.

Divide the batter among the muffin cups and bake until the muffins are browned and a toothpick comes out clean, 20 to 25 minutes.

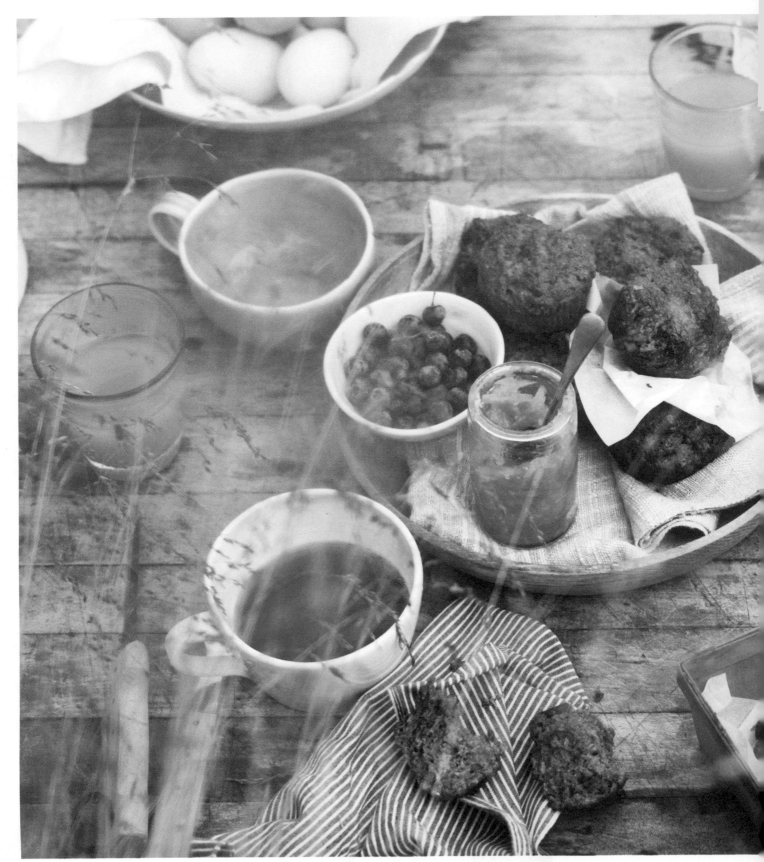

In basket, Sweet Potato + Five-Spice Muffins (page 41); *on plate at top*, "Buttermilk" Waffles (page 38);
and, *at far right*, Momo's Special Turkey Bacon (page 224)

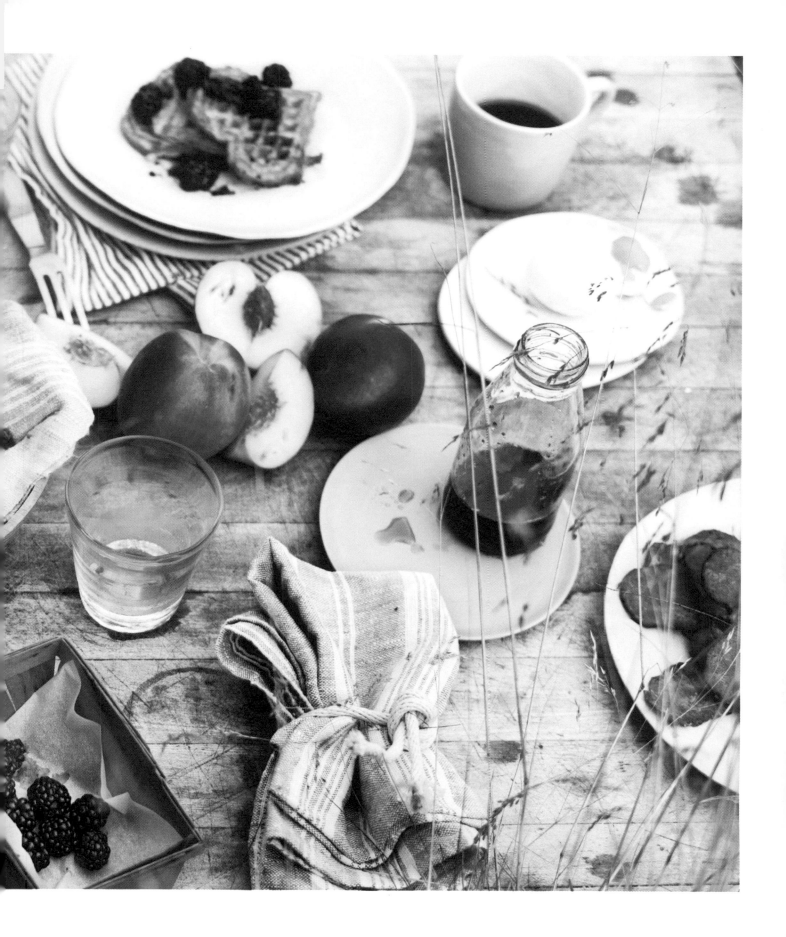

BANANA-DATE MUFFINS

These muffins strike a comforting chord for people who adore banana bread (which seems to be everyone). Without compromising health, flavor, or texture, these are studded with sweet dates and topped with crunchy pumpkin seeds and are the best-ever use for overripe bananas.

Makes a dozen muffins

Ⓥ Vegan

2 cups gluten-free flour plus 1 tablespoon (if the
       flour doesn't include xanthan gum, add 1
       teaspoon)
2 teaspoons baking powder
2 teaspoons baking soda
A pinch of sea salt
2 overripe bananas, mashed
½ cup extra virgin olive oil
⅔ cup good-quality maple syrup
⅔ cup unsweetened almond milk
2 teaspoons pure vanilla extract
½ pitted and chopped cup dried dates
       (about 6 large dates)
¼ cup roughly chopped pumpkin seeds, plus
       3 tablespoons for the tops of the muffins

Preheat the oven to 400°F. Line a 12-cup muffin tin with paper liners.

Whisk together the 2 cups of flour, the baking powder, baking soda, and salt in a bowl. In a separate bowl, whisk together the bananas, olive oil, maple syrup, almond milk, and vanilla. Thoroughly combine the dry and the wet ingredients. Toss the dates and the ¼ cup of chopped pumpkin seeds with the extra tablespoon of flour (this keeps them from sinking to the bottom of the muffins) and fold them into the batter with a rubber spatula. Evenly divide the batter among the muffin cups and sprinkle each muffin with a pinch of the extra pumpkin seeds.

Bake until the muffins are browned and a toothpick comes out clean, 20 to 25 minutes.

SCRAMBLED TOFU

I like this as part of a savory breakfast alongside Go-To Black Beans (see page 275), Pickled Jalapeños (see page 280), and sliced avocado, but it also works well as a vegetarian taco filling.

Serves 4

Ⓥ Vegan Ⓟ Protein-Packed

3 tablespoons extra virgin olive oil
2 garlic cloves, finely chopped
1 teaspoon cumin
A 14-ounce box firm tofu, drained and crumbled
Coarse sea salt
Freshly ground black pepper

Heat the olive oil in a large nonstick pan over high heat and cook the garlic and cumin, stirring, until fragrant, not even 1 minute. Add the tofu, turn down the heat to medium, and cook, stirring now and then, until just beginning to brown, about 5 minutes. Season to taste with salt and pepper and serve.

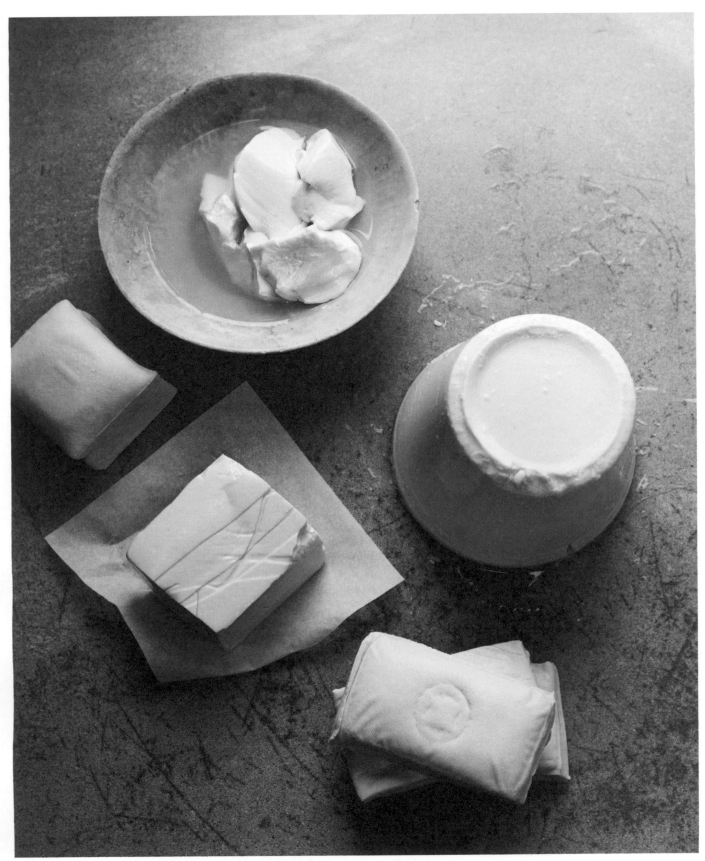

Various types of tofu

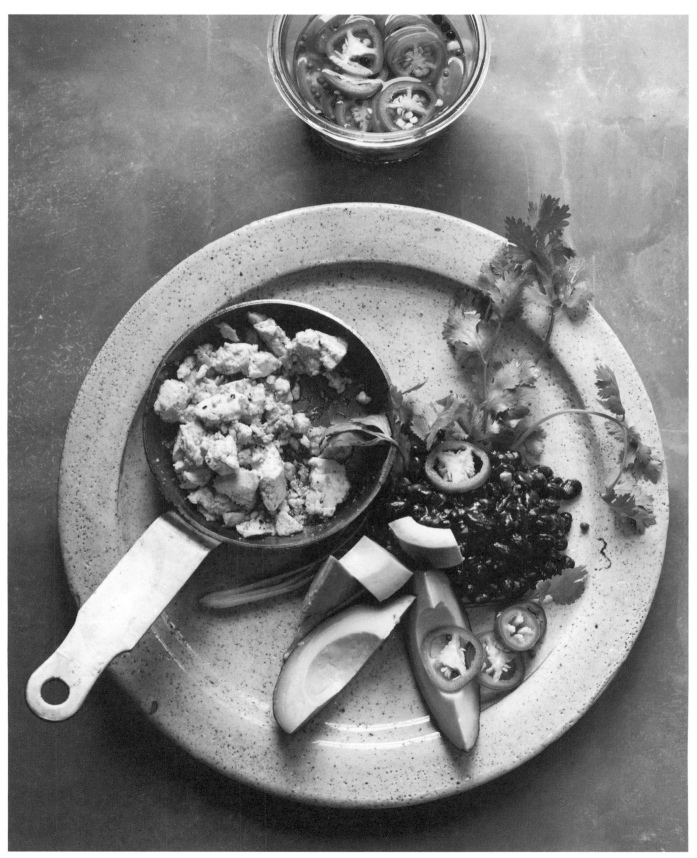

Scrambled Tofu (page 47) plated with avocados, Pickled Jalapeños (page 280), and Go-To Black Beans (page 275)

AN ACTUALLY GOOD EGG-WHITE OMELET, TWO WAYS

This is what to make in the morning if your boyfriend is a body builder. Or you want him to look like one. We got the idea to partially whip the egg whites from a Jean-Georges Vongerichten recipe: that's the secret to the pleasing texture.

Each version serves 1

Ⓟ Protein-Packed (both versions)

HUEVOS RANCHEROS VERSION

4 chicken or duck eggs
Coarse sea salt
Freshly ground black pepper
3 tablespoons roughly torn cilantro
Cooking spray
½ cup warm Go-To Black Beans (see page 275)
1 lime
Cholula Hot Sauce
A few Pickled Jalapeños (see page 280) and
    sliced avocado for serving, if desired

Separate the egg whites from their yolks (reserve the yolks for another use). Whisk the egg whites in a bowl with a pinch of salt and a few grinds of black pepper until they're foamy. Stir in half the cilantro.

Spray a small nonstick pan with cooking spray and set it over medium heat. Add the egg whites and cook until they just begin to set on the bottom, about 1 minute. Cover the pan and cook 1 minute more, or until the top of the egg whites is set and opaque. Fold one half over the other into a half-moon shape and slide onto a plate alongside the black beans. Grate a bit of the zest from the lime on top of the omelet, sprinkle with the remaining cilantro, and shake a few drops of Cholula on top. Serve with a few Pickled Jalapeños and some sliced avocado if you like.

SPINACH + MUSHROOM VERSION

1 tablespoon extra virgin olive oil
1 garlic clove, minced
12 button or crimini mushrooms, thinly sliced
¼ yellow onion, very thinly sliced
2 handfuls of baby spinach
Coarse sea salt
Freshly ground black pepper
4 chicken or duck eggs
Cooking spray

Heat the olive oil in a nonstick skillet over medium heat. Add the garlic and cook, stirring, just until fragrant, about 1 minute. Add the mushrooms and stir them into the garlic until they start to soften, about 1 more minute. Add the onion and cook until all the vegetables are soft and just beginning to brown, about 10 minutes. Add the spinach and stir until it wilts, just about 1 minute. Season the mixture to taste with salt and pepper. Set the mixture aside.

Meanwhile, separate the egg whites from their yolks (reserve the yolks for another use). Whisk the egg whites in a bowl with a pinch of salt and a few grinds of black pepper until they're foamy.

Spray a small nonstick pan with cooking spray and set it over medium heat. Add the egg whites and cook until they just begin to set on the bottom, about 1 minute. Cover the pan and cook 1 minute more, or until the top of the egg whites is set and opaque. Top half of the omelet with the reserved spinach and mushroom mixture. Fold the other half over to form a half-moon shape and slide the omelet onto a plate. Serve immediately.

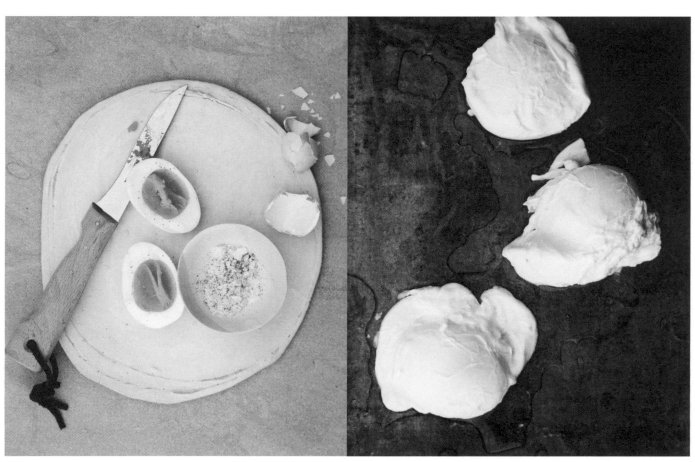

An Egg, Three Ways (page 278) *From left to right*, a hard-boiled egg; poached eggs; an olive oil–fried egg

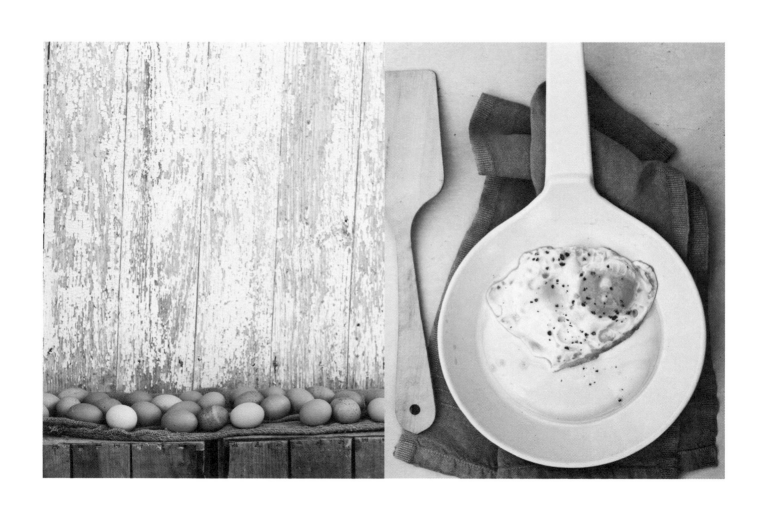

SALADS + A FEW GREAT DRESSINGS

My absolute favorite thing to eat for lunch, bar none, is a salad. Not a few greens on a plate (that's a side!), but a delicious medley of beautiful, filling, harmonious ingredients. The more we focus on health, the more salads become a great main course option. What better way to get all your veggies and protein in endless combinations without compromising taste or health? The key to any mouthwatering salad is the dressing, and in this chapter we collect an array of incredibly flavorful ones that are easy to make and could transform even plain old lettuce into something special.

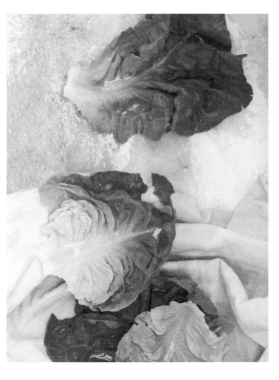
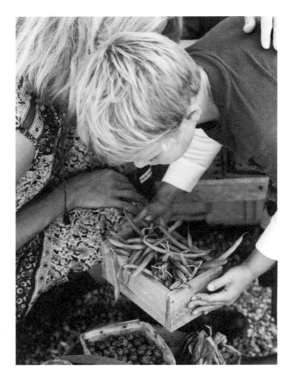
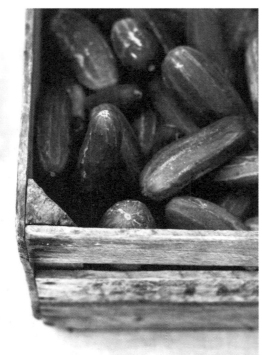
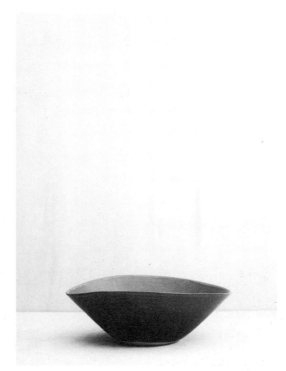

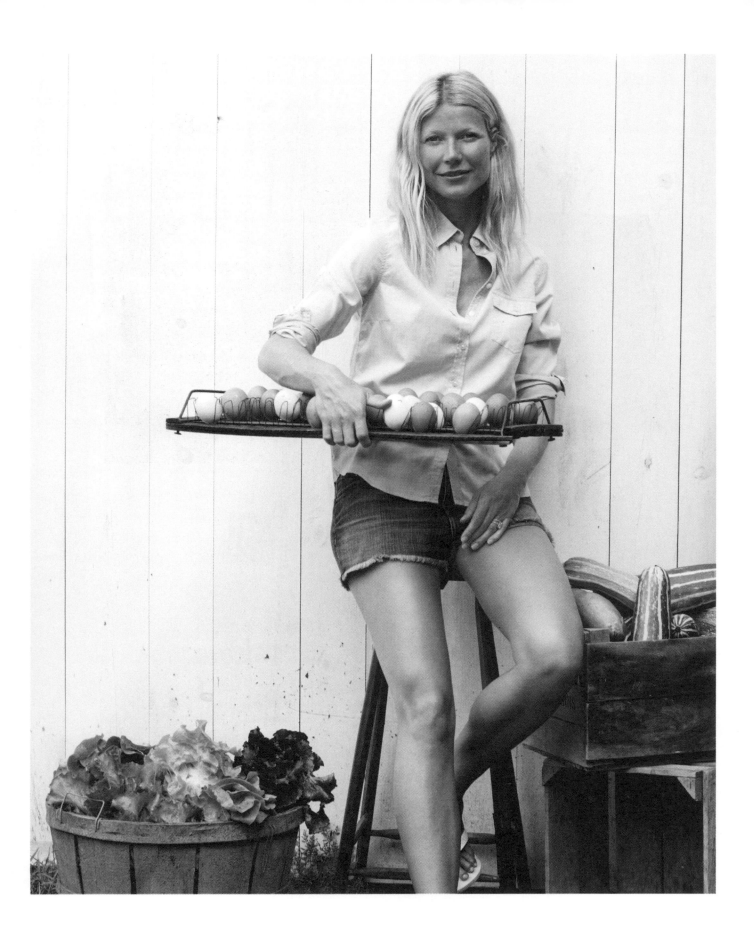

MEXICAN CHOPPED SALAD WITH MEXICAN GREEN GODDESS DRESSING

Mexican flavors are among my favorites in the world, but when you're eliminating processed corn and gluten, you lose all your tortilla options. Not to fear—this delicious salad is full of Mexican tastes and so filling that you won't miss the chips or wrap at all.

Serves 4

V Vegan **P** Protein-Packed

2 fresh ears of corn, shucked
2 hearts of romaine, finely shredded (about
    5 cups of lettuce)
Mexican Green Goddess Dressing
½ cup cooked black beans (use half a drained and
    rinsed 14-ounce can)
½ cup chopped tomatoes (or ½ cup halved cherry
    tomatoes)
4 scallions, white and light green parts only, very
    thinly sliced
1 ripe avocado, diced
¼ cup roughly chopped cilantro

Steam or grill the corn until it's cooked through. When it's cool enough to handle, slice the kernels off the cobs and set them aside (discard the cobs).

Place the lettuce in a large bowl and dress it with ¼ cup of the dressing so it has just a light coating. Divide the lettuce among 4 plates or place it on a large platter. Over the lettuce, evenly scatter the beans, tomatoes, scallions, avocado, cilantro, and reserved corn. Drizzle each portion with another tablespoon or 2 of the dressing and serve immediately, with the remaining dressing on the side if you or your guests like your salad more heavily dressed.

MEXICAN GREEN GODDESS DRESSING

V Vegan if you use Vegenaise

This makes a lot—don't worry, you'll use it.

Makes 1¼ cups

⅔ cup sheep's or goat's milk yogurt or Vegenaise
¼ cup cilantro
2 scallions, white and light green parts only,
    roughly chopped
¼ cup freshly squeezed lime juice
½ green jalapeño, roughly chopped (or use more
    or less, whatever you prefer!)
½ cup extra virgin olive oil
½ teaspoon coarse sea salt
1 tablespoon raw honey or xylitol

Combine all the ingredients in a powerful blender and blitz until completely smooth.

Keeps well in a jar in the fridge for up to a week.

LEE'S CHOPPED VIETNAMESE SALAD

Lee Gross is a (mostly) macrobiotic chef I have known
and worked with at various times over the past decade.
He taught me about macrobiotics around the time my
father became ill and I was hell-bent on the family's
eating better. Lee was trained by Michio Kushi at the
Kushi Institute in Becket, Massachusetts, and at Johnson
& Wales University in Rhode Island, and his food
beautifully fuses healthy and delicious. He has taught
me a world of food knowledge that I apply all the time.
This healthy, quick salad has great crunch and lots
of refreshing flavors. It's wonderful on its own and also
takes well to simply prepared proteins—grilled fish,
shrimp, chicken, and tofu are all great with it.

Serves 4

4 large bok choy leaves, rough bottoms
     discarded, stems cut on the bias into ¼-inch
     pieces, and leaves shredded
4 big leaves Napa cabbage, shredded
1 bunch of watercress (discard thick stems),
     roughly chopped
1 large carrot, peeled and cut into matchsticks
Leaves from about 8 sprigs each of basil, mint,
     and cilantro, roughly chopped
½ small cucumber, thinly sliced on the bias
1 red Thai chili (or more…or less), thinly sliced
½ cup roasted, salted peanuts or cashews,
     roughly chopped
Vietnamese Dressing

Toss the bok choy, cabbage, watercress, carrot, herbs,
cucumber, chili, and ¼ cup of the nuts together with
enough dressing to coat. Serve sprinkled with the
remaining nuts.

VIETNAMESE DRESSING

A perfect balance of hot, sour, salty, and sweet,
this dressing is a flavor knockout. Also a great dip
for summer rolls.

Makes about ¾ cup

¼ cup freshly squeezed lime juice
1 tablespoon rice wine vinegar
2 teaspoons soy sauce
¼ cup fish sauce
¼ teaspoon sea salt
¼ teaspoon hot toasted sesame oil
2 tablespoons raw honey or xylitol
1 teaspoon minced garlic
1 teaspoon minced fresh ginger
2 tablespoons finely diced red onion or shallot

Mix everything together. Keeps well in a jar in the fridge
for up to a week.

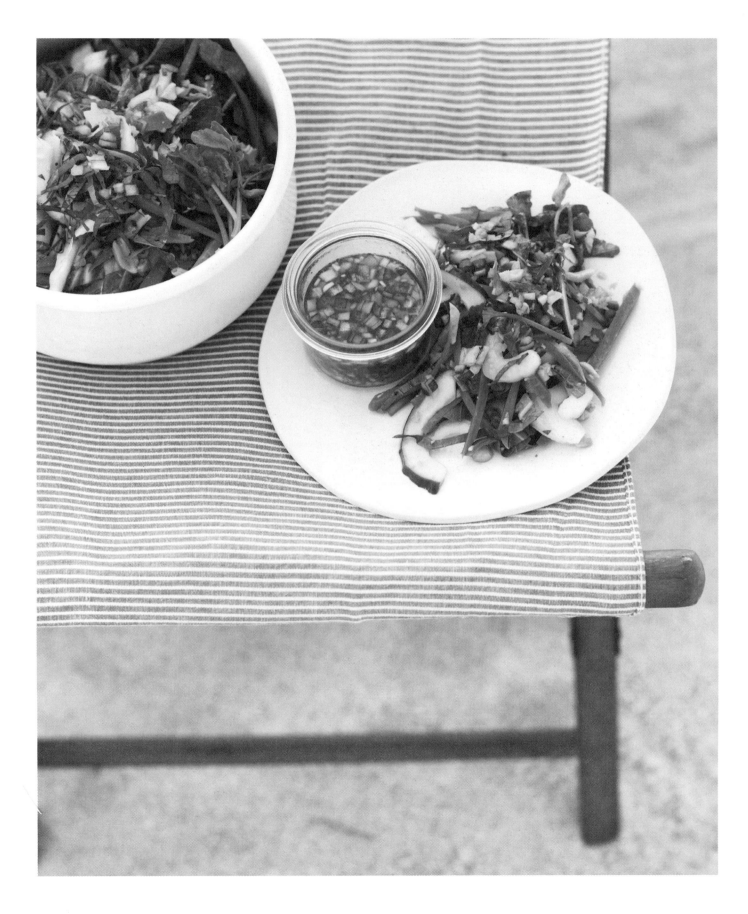

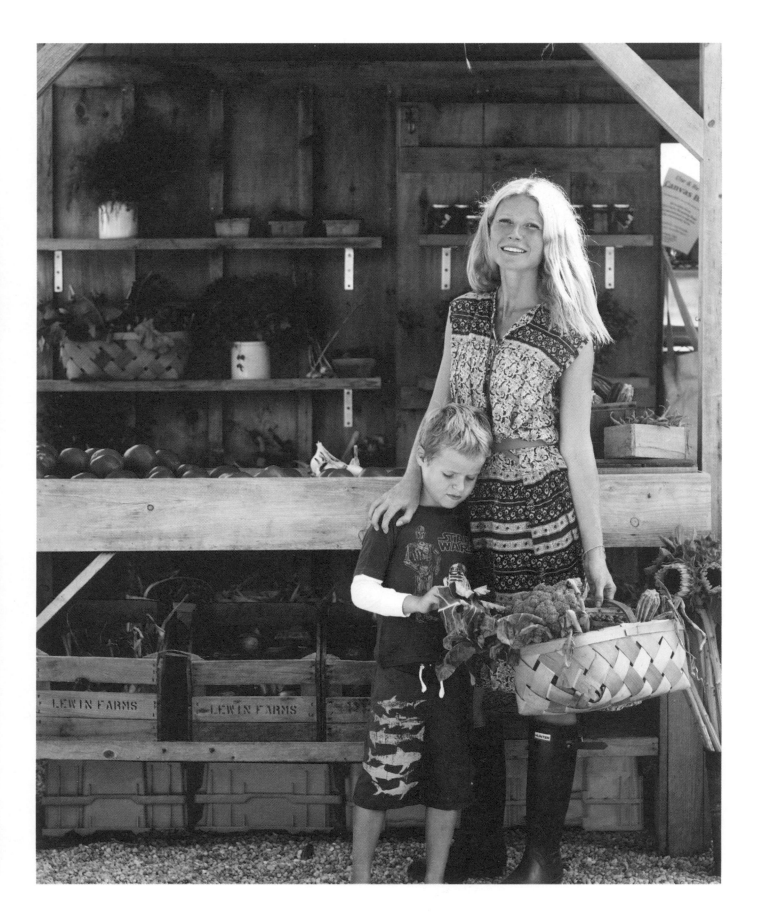

POWER CHOPPED SALAD WITH CREAMY PARSLEY DRESSING

This is one of my faves. I like to serve it in the summertime when tomatoes are in season. It's a great vegetarian option that still has loads of protein.

Serves 4

Ⓟ Protein-Packed

2 hearts of romaine, finely shredded
2 handfuls of baby arugula, roughly chopped
Creamy Parsley Dressing
A 14-ounce can chickpeas, rinsed and drained
2 vine-ripened tomatoes, diced
2 cooked beets, peeled and diced
4 hard-boiled eggs (see A Hard-Boiled Egg, page 278), peeled and quartered

Place the romaine and arugula in a large bowl and stir to combine with ¼ cup of the dressing so the lettuces have just a light coating. Divide the mixture among 4 plates or place it on a large platter. Over the top of the lettuce, evenly scatter the chickpeas, tomatoes, beets, and hard-boiled eggs. Drizzle each portion with another tablespoon or 2 of the dressing and serve immediately, with the remaining dressing on the side if you or your guests like your salad more heavily dressed.

CREAMY PARSLEY DRESSING

Ⓥ Vegan

Makes about 1¼ cups

Leaves from 1 bunch of Italian parsley
    (about 1 cup)
3 tablespoons white wine vinegar
¼ cup extra virgin olive oil
¼ cup Vegenaise
3 tablespoons water
1 tablespoon xylitol
½ teaspoon coarse sea salt
¼ teaspoon freshly ground pepper

Combine all the ingredients in a powerful blender and blitz until completely pureed.

Keeps well in a jar in the fridge for up to a week.

NY STREET VENDOR SALAD WITH YOGURT-TAHINI DRESSING

This is a flavor-packed salad that's all about the dressing (isn't it always?). It's especially good alongside Tandoori Turkey Kabobs (see page 107) or Middle Eastern Turkey Burgers (see page 108).

Serves 4

Ⓥ Vegan

1 large head of romaine or 3 heads of Little Gem
    lettuce, chopped
A handful of cherry tomatoes, halved
½ English cucumber, peeled and diced
⅓ red onion, very thinly sliced or shaved on
    a mandoline
Yogurt-Tahini Dressing

Place the lettuce in a large bowl and stir to combine with ¼ cup of the dressing so it's just lightly coated. Divide the lettuce among 4 plates or place it on a large platter. Over the lettuce, evenly scatter the tomatoes, cucumber, and onion. Drizzle each portion with another tablespoon or 2 of the dressing and serve immediately, with the remaining dressing on the side if you or your guests like your salad more heavily dressed.

YOGURT-TAHINI DRESSING

Ⓥ Vegan (if you use Vegenaise)

Makes 1 cup

2 tablespoons tahini
¼ cup boiling water
½ small garlic clove, finely minced
½ cup plain sheep's or goat's milk yogurt or
    Vegenaise
3 tablespoons freshly squeezed lemon juice
¼ cup extra virgin olive oil
½ teaspoon coarse sea salt
¼ teaspoon freshly ground black pepper

Whisk the tahini and water together until completely smooth. Whisk in the remaining ingredients. That's it.

Keeps well in a jar in the fridge for up to a week.

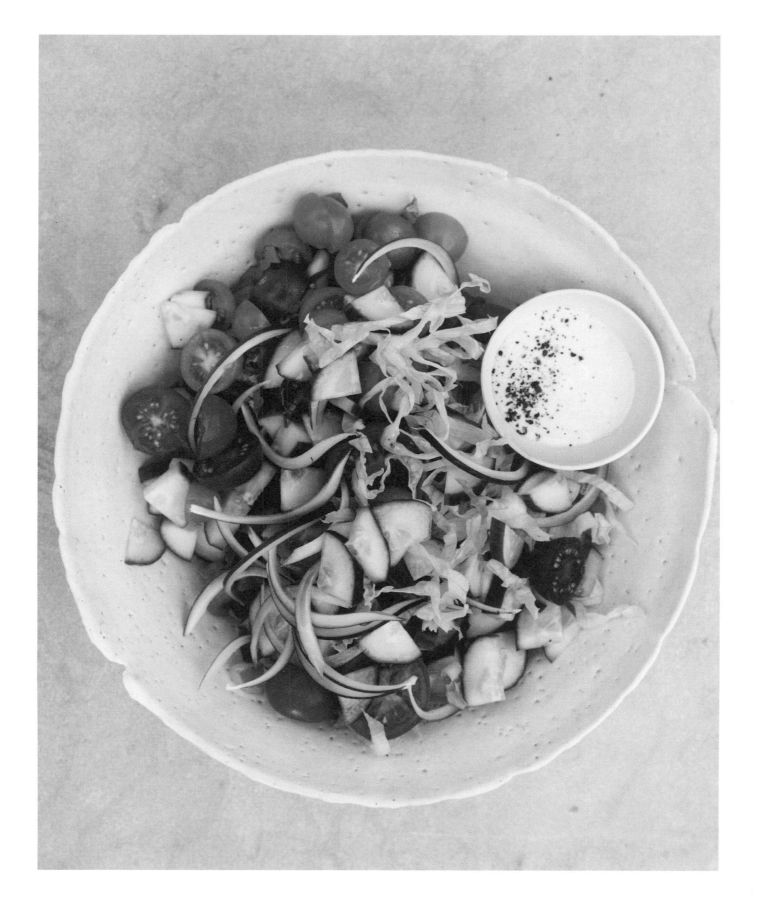

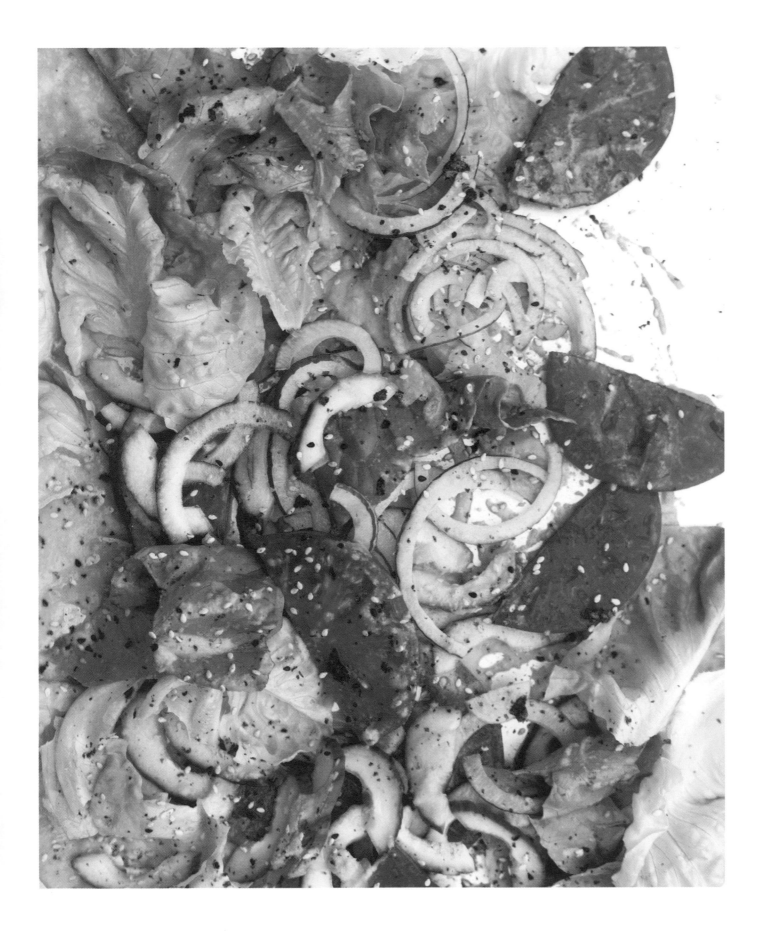

JAPANESE RESTAURANT–STYLE SALAD WITH CARROT-GINGER DRESSING

I first developed this salad and salad dressing recipe for my website, GOOP.com, but have tweaked it just slightly and doubled everything, since there never seemed to be enough.

Serves 4

Ⓥ Vegan

1 head of Bibb lettuce, torn
1 ripe tomato, sliced
½ cucumber, sliced
½ red onion, thinly sliced
⅔ cup Carrot-Ginger Dressing
2 teaspoons Seaweed Sesame Sprinkle
    (see page 287)

Put the lettuce into a salad bowl and top with the tomato, cucumber, and red onion. Drizzle with plenty of the dressing, sprinkle with the Seaweed Sesame Sprinkle, and serve immediately.

CARROT-GINGER DRESSING

This keeps well in a jar in the fridge for up to a week—for a satisfying snack, put a spoonful of the dressing into half an avocado and go to town Kids also really like this, and if yours don't go for salad, use it as a dip for sliced peppers, steamed green beans or broccoli, or whatever vegetables they're into.

Ⓥ Vegan

Makes 2½ cups

2 carrots, peeled and roughly chopped
2 shallots, peeled and roughly chopped
¼ cup roughly chopped fresh ginger
2 tablespoons sweet white miso paste
¼ cup rice vinegar
2 tablespoons light raw honey or xylitol
2 tablespoons toasted sesame oil
½ cup grapeseed oil
¼ cup water
½ teaspoon coarse sea salt
½ teaspoon freshly ground black pepper

Puree everything together in a powerful blender until absolutely smooth.

SPANISH CHOPPED SALAD WITH TUNA + PIQUILLOS WITH SPANISH SALAD DRESSING

Julia here. Gwyneth and I met each other in Spain while she was shooting *Spain...On the Road Again*, a public television show about Spanish food and culture. Since then, we've swooned together over tins of olive oil–packed anchovies and tuna, smoky pimentón, and heavy pours of sherry vinegar. This salad, full of incredibly bold flavors, is totally satisfying and full of protein while still being terrifically good for you.

Serves 4

Ⓟ Protein-Packed

A 14-ounce can chickpeas, rinsed and drained
2 tablespoons extra virgin olive oil
1 teaspoon sweet pimentón (or use the hot
　　version, often labeled *picante*, if you want a
　　bit of a kick)
Coarse sea salt
1 large head of butter/Bibb/Boston lettuce (a rose
　　is a rose...), carefully washed and dried
1 recipe Spanish Salad Dressing
3 scallions, white and light green parts only,
　　finely sliced
2 jarred roasted piquillo peppers, thinly sliced
8 ounces olive oil–packed tuna, oil drained off
　　and saved for another use
2 tablespoons roughly chopped Italian parsley

Preheat the oven to 425°F and line a sheet pan with a piece of parchment paper.

Place the chickpeas on the prepared pan, drizzle them with the olive oil, and sprinkle them with the pimentón and a large pinch of salt. Use your hands to move the chickpeas around and get them evenly coated. Roast the chickpeas, stirring now and then, until they're dark brown and a little bit dried and crunchy, 15 to 20 minutes. Set them aside to cool.

Meanwhile, tear the lettuce into bite-sized pieces and place them in a large mixing bowl. Gently stir the lettuce with half the dressing so it's just lightly coated. Place the lettuce on a large platter and evenly sprinkle it with the roasted chickpeas, scallions, and piquillo peppers. Using your hands, break the tuna into big flakes over the salad. Evenly spoon the rest of the dressing over the salad, sprinkle the whole thing with the parsley, and dig in.

SPANISH SALAD DRESSING

This dressing uses two signature Spanish ingredients in unexpected ways. Membrillo paste, often served alongside Manchego cheese, provides some sweetness, and the olive oil that the anchovies come packed in is embraced as its own ingredient.

Makes ⅔ cup

2 tablespoons membrillo (quince) paste or
　　good-quality raw honey
¼ cup sherry vinegar
2 tablespoons olive oil from a jar or can of
　　anchovies (look up *anchovy* in the index
　　for tons of ideas about what to do with
　　the leftover anchovies)
⅓ cup extra virgin olive oil
Coarse sea salt
Freshly ground black pepper

Combine the membrillo, vinegar, and anchovy oil in a powerful blender and blitz until totally combined. With the machine running, slowly add the olive oil. Season to taste with salt and pepper.

Keeps well in the a jar in the fridge for up to a week.

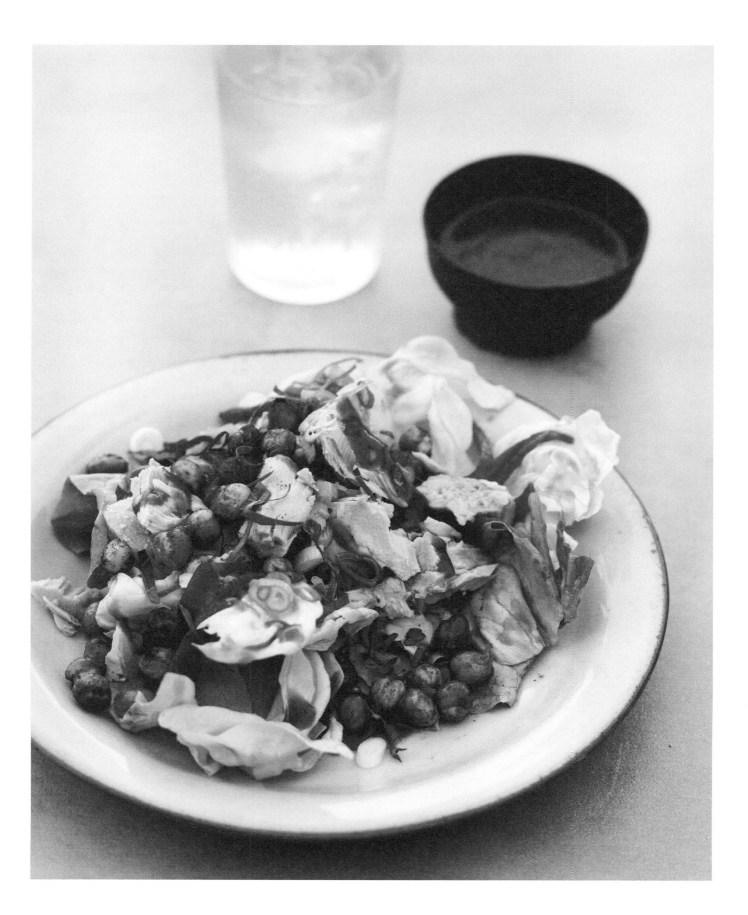

MANGO + AVOCADO SALAD WITH BALSAMIC-LIME VINAIGRETTE

So beautiful and so simple to prepare, this salad is also delicious with a few slices of heirloom tomatoes in the summertime in addition to mangoes (if you're NOT avoiding nightshades because of inflammation, etc....).

Serves 4

E Elimination Diet **V** Vegan

2 ripe mangoes, peeled, pitted, and thinly sliced
2 ripe avocados, peeled, pitted, and thinly sliced
Coarse sea salt
1 batch Balsamic-Lime Vinaigrette
A small handful of fresh basil leaves

Alternate slices of mango and avocado on a serving platter and scatter with a pinch of sea salt. Drizzle with the Balsamic-Lime vinaigrette; tear the basil leaves and sprinkle them over the top. Serve immediately.

BALSAMIC-LIME VINAIGRETTE

Makes about ⅔ cup

E Elimination Diet **V** Vegan

2 tablespoons balsamic vinegar
2 tablespoons brown rice syrup
1 tablespoon freshly squeezed lime juice
¼ cup plus 2 tablespoons extra virgin olive oil
Coarse sea salt
Freshly ground pepper

Whisk the vinegar, brown rice syrup, and lime juice together in a mixing bowl. Slowly whisk in the olive oil and season to taste with salt and pepper.

Keeps well in a jar in the fridge for up to a week.

ARUGULA SALAD WITH ROASTED BEETS, SQUASH + SHALLOTS WITH APPLE CIDER VINAIGRETTE

Apple cider vinegar is all the rage with health nuts, for good reasons—it's full of enzymes and potassium, it's great for digestion, it's said to be good for the skin and immune system; it's even good for soothing sore throats. From a cooking perspective, I love its fall flavor and find that it's a natural complement to beets, butternut squash, and shallots. The maple syrup adds another layer of autumnal yum.

Serves 4

Ⓥ Vegan

2 large beets, peeled and cut into ½-inch cubes
     (about 2 cups)
1 small butternut squash, peeled, seeded, and
     cut into ½-inch cubes (about 3 cups)
6 large shallots, peeled and roughly chopped
Extra virgin olive oil
Coarse sea salt
4 ounces baby arugula
½ cup toasted pumpkin seeds

Preheat the oven to 425°F and line a sheet pan with parchment paper.

Combine the beets, squash, and shallots on the prepared pan and drizzle them with 3 tablespoons of olive oil. Sprinkle with a generous pinch of salt and roast, stirring now and then, until cooked through and nicely caramelized, 30 to 35 minutes.

Place the arugula in a large bowl and coat with half the dressing. Lay the dressed arugula on a serving platter, then place the roasted vegetables in the bowl that you dressed the arugula in and coat them with the remainder of the dressing. Artfully arrange the vegetables on top of the arugula, sprinkle the whole thing with the toasted pumpkin seeds, and serve immediately.

APPLE CIDER VINAIGRETTE

Makes ¾ cup

Ⓥ Vegan

1 tablespoon Dijon mustard
3 tablespoons apple cider vinegar
2 tablespoons good-quality maple syrup
½ cup olive oil
Coarse sea salt
Freshly ground black pepper

Whisk together the mustard, vinegar, and maple syrup in a mixing bowl. While whisking, slowly drizzle in the olive oil. Season the vinaigrette to taste with salt and pepper.

Keeps well in a jar in the fridge for up to a week.

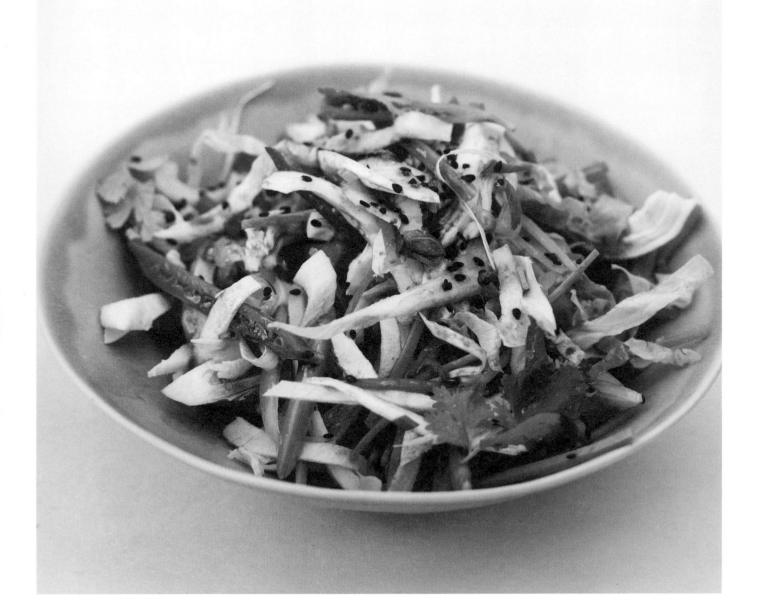

CHINESE CHICKEN SALAD

This recipe makes more than enough dressing, but whatever's left over is great on grilled fish or chicken or on a bowl of brown rice. The preparation goes quickly if you prep the dressing and all your vegetables while the chicken steams. The steaming liquid can be strained and enjoyed as a light, wonderful broth.

Serves 2 generously

(P) Protein-Packed

4 coin-sized pieces fresh ginger, crushed with the side of your knife
2 garlic cloves, crushed with the side of your knife
6 scallions, 2 bruised with the side of your knife and the other 4 finely sliced lengthwise
½ star anise
1 teaspoon Chinese five-spice powder
2 chicken breasts on the bone, skin removed
1 head of Little Gem lettuce (or 1 heart of romaine), core discarded, finely shredded
1 head of green endive, core discarded, finely shredded
1 head of red endive, core discarded, finely shredded (or just use another green endive)
A handful of snow peas, thinly sliced lengthwise
1 carrot, peeled and cut into matchsticks
3 tablespoons cilantro, roughly chopped
A little bit of freshly minced red chili (optional)
A big pinch of toasted black sesame seeds
Chinese Chicken Salad Dressing

Bring a few cups of water to a boil in a large wok or pot along with the ginger, the garlic, the 2 bruised scallions, the star anise, and the Chinese five-spice powder. Turn the heat down and let the mixture simmer for 5 minutes. Set up a steamer (bamboo or whatever you've got) above the fragrant mixture and steam the chicken breasts for 45 minutes. Set the chicken aside until it's cool enough to handle, then shred the meat with your fingers, discarding the bones.

Combine the shredded chicken with the 4 sliced scallions, the Little Gem, the endive, the snow peas, the carrot, the cilantro, the chili (if using), and the black sesame seeds and stir to combine with as much of the dressing as you like.

CHINESE CHICKEN SALAD DRESSING

Makes about a cup

(V) Vegan

3 tablespoons Lee's Hoisin Sauce (page 275)
⅓ cup cold-pressed, untoasted sesame oil (or extra virgin olive oil)
1 tablespoon brown rice vinegar
¼ cup water

Whisk everything together. Keeps well in a jar in the fridge for up to a week.

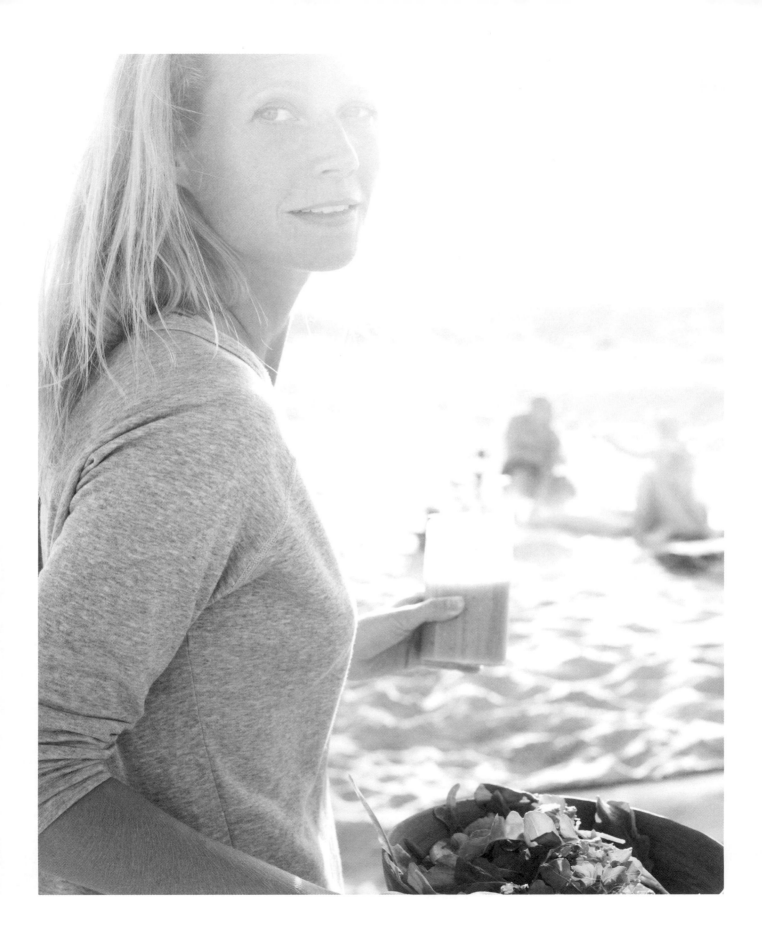

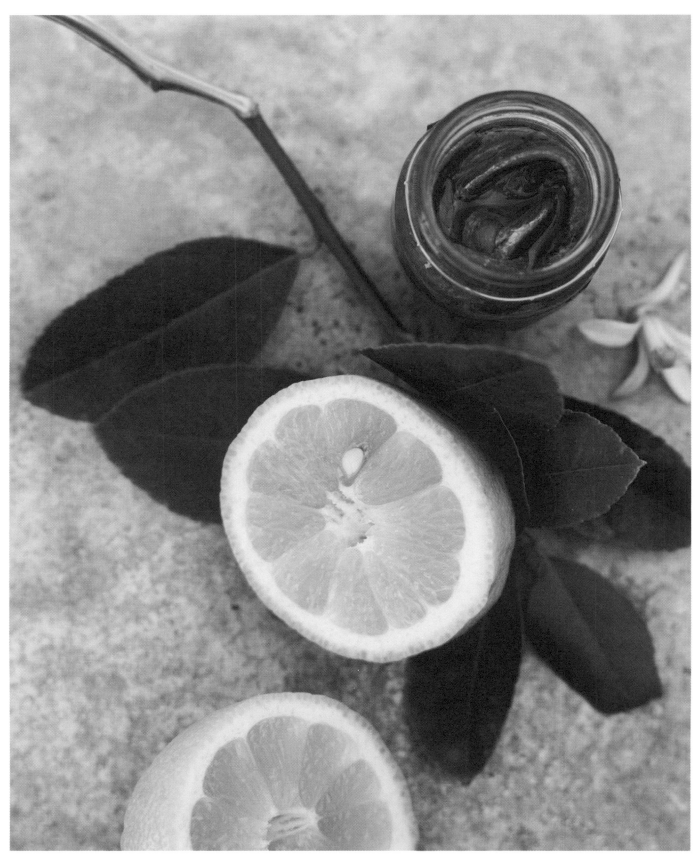

Some ingredients for Anchovy + Lemon Dressing (page 74)

ANCHOVY + LEMON DRESSING

This stuff's like money in the bank. Keep a jar in the fridge—use it to dress arugula, finely sliced radicchio, escarole, or any bitter green. Cook down greens—kale, spinach, the leafy tops of beets, the greens that hug a cauliflower, which you normally throw away—in olive oil with garlic and red chili and then drizzle a few spoonfuls of this over them. Roast a piece of fish and give it a bath in this dressing. You really can't go wrong.

Makes 1 generous cup

E Elimination Diet

8 olive oil–packed anchovies (preferably Spanish)
5 tablespoons freshly squeezed lemon juice
¾ cup extra virgin olive oil
Coarse sea salt
Freshly ground black pepper

Combine the anchovies and lemon juice in a powerful blender and blitz until totally combined. With the machine running, slowly add the olive oil. Season to taste with salt and pepper.

Keeps well in a jar in the fridge for up to a week.

GREEN GODDESS DRESSING

Green Goddess is the perfect name for this heavenly dressing, which elevates any salad or crudité. It's gorgeously creamy yet dairy free.

Makes 1¼ cups

Ⓥ Vegan

10 large basil leaves
3 tablespoons chopped chives
2 tablespoons cilantro (leaves from about 5 sprigs)
¼ cup Italian parsley (leaves from about 5 sprigs)
Leaves from 1 sprig of tarragon
2 scallions, white and light green parts only,
    roughly chopped
½ ripe avocado
¼ cup Vegenaise
2 tablespoons raw honey or xylitol
2 tablespoons white wine vinegar
Juice of 1 lemon (about ¼ cup)
3 tablespoons extra virgin olive oil
¼ cup water
½ teaspoon coarse sea salt
¼ teaspoon freshly ground black pepper

Combine all the ingredients in a powerful blender and blitz until completely pureed.

Keeps well in a jar in the fridge for up to a week.

OLD BAY RANCH DRESSING

This dressing combines the classic flavors of old-school ranch dressing with Old Bay seasoning, one of our most beloved ingredients. This is delicious on grilled or roasted fish or Best Gluten-Free Fish Fingers (see page 234) and is also a great dip for raw or steamed vegetables.

Makes ½ cup

Ⓥ Vegan

½ cup Vegenaise
2 teaspoons freshly squeezed lemon juice
1 teaspoon Old Bay seasoning
1 garlic clove, finely minced
1 tablespoon finely chopped chives

Combine all the ingredients in a bowl and whisk together.

Keeps well in a jar in the fridge for up to a week.

SOUPS

Soup is a fantastic thing to eat when you're cleaning up your food program. It is (mostly) hot and filling, oh so comforting, and a terrific way to pack nutrition into your meal. If you eat chicken, a great chicken stock serves as a wonderful base for flavor in soups. A nutritionist once told me that stock made from bones is a good way to strengthen your own! I come from a long line of Jewish cooking mamas, and I've got the chicken soup recipe to prove it. My grandmother's father was a chicken farmer on Long Island back in the day; so needless to say, chicken soup is in my blood. My version (page 82) is on the stove all winter; when I want to change it up, I take out the kale and carrots and add some fish sauce, chili, garlic, lemongrass, and lime (with whatever veggies are around) and I have a spicy Thai chicken soup that's a real cold buster. If you're vegetarian or vegan, a great veggie stock builds flavor underneath any vegetable soup you can think of. In this chapter you'll find very healthy, filling, very clean soups to help your diet/detox/ clean living plan be just as tasty as can be.

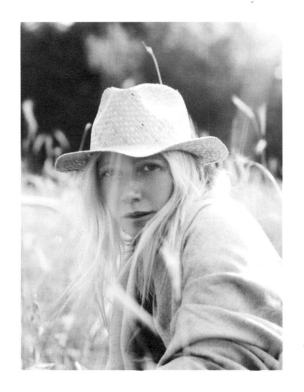
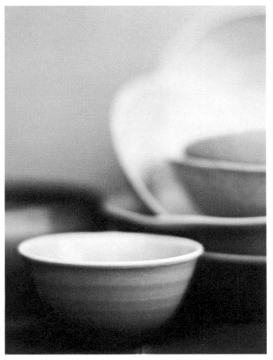
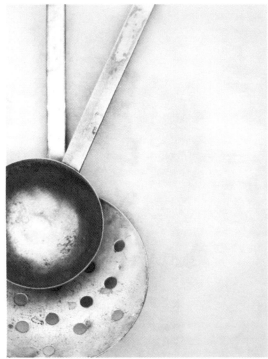
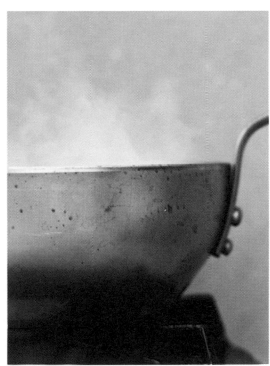

BROCCOLI + ARUGULA SOUP
(AKA ANY-VEGETABLE SOUP)

This is a clean, basic approach to soup that showcases the vegetables. You can vary this recipe with anything—peas and basil, zucchini, carrots and ginger. In this case, broccoli is made a bit more dynamic with a handful of peppery arugula. When you're detoxing and drinking lots of juices and smoothies, it's a nice change to have something warm. It's easy to double this recipe, so you can make it once and eat it twice.

Serves 2

E Elimination Diet **V** Vegan

1 tablespoon extra virgin olive oil
1 garlic clove, thinly sliced
½ yellow onion, roughly diced
1 head of broccoli, cut into small florets
    (about ⅔ pound)
2½ cups water
¼ teaspoon coarse sea salt
¼ teaspoon freshly ground black pepper
¾ cup arugula (watercress would be good, too)
½ lemon

Heat the olive oil in a medium nonstick saucepan over medium heat. Add the garlic and onion and sauté for just 1 minute, or until fragrant. Add the broccoli and cook for 4 minutes, or until bright green. Add the water, salt, and pepper; bring to a boil, lower the heat, and cover. Cook for 8 minutes, or until the broccoli is just tender. Pour the soup into a powerful blender and puree with the arugula until quite smooth. (Be very careful when blending hot liquids. Start slowly and work in batches if necessary—you don't want the steam to blow the lid off.) Pour into serving bowls and squeeze the ½ lemon equally over each.

MISO SOUP WITH WATERCRESS

You can make the broth early in the week and add the miso as you eat. Also, you can eat this plain, or with the watercress, or bulk it up with other thinly sliced vegetables (mushrooms, zucchini, carrots, etc.). The bonito, flakes of dried tuna, are available at Asian grocery stores and add tremendous depth of flavor, but feel free to skip them if you're vegetarian or vegan. The wakame, a dried seaweed, is also readily available at Asian grocery stores.

Serves 4

E Elimination Diet **V** Vegan (without the bonito flakes)

6 cups water
Small handful dried bonito flakes
3 dried shiitake mushrooms
A 4-inch piece of dried wakame
6 tablespoons miso paste (whatever kind you
    like—sweet white miso makes for a nice,
    light soup, while aged barley miso gives a
    full, robust flavor)
2 cups watercress, washed

Heat the water in a small soup pot. When bubbles form around the edge, add the bonito. Turn the heat down and simmer for 2 minutes. Turn off the heat and let the broth sit for 5 minutes. Strain the broth into a clean pot, discarding the bonito. Add the shiitakes and wakame to the broth and simmer over low heat for 20 minutes. Remove the shiitakes and wakame. Discard the thick stems from the mushrooms, thinly slice the caps, and slip them back into the broth. Chop the wakame into small pieces, discarding any thick pieces of stem, and return to the pot.

In a small bowl, combine the miso paste with a bit of the broth and whisk to blend. Pour the mixture back into the pot and let the soup simmer, being careful not to let it boil. Add the watercress at the last minute just to wilt it, and serve.

BEET, FENNEL + APPLE SOUP

An homage to borscht, this stunningly pink soup is best in the early fall, when the last of summer's beets overlap with the first new apples. We have apple trees, so we love this recipe. It's great topped with a spoonful of goat's milk yogurt mixed with a spoonful of horseradish.

Serves 4

E Elimination Diet **V** Vegan

2 tablespoons extra virgin olive oil
1 fennel bulb, green parts discarded, white parts diced
1 yellow onion, diced
2 garlic cloves, finely minced
Coarse sea salt
3 medium beets, peeled and roughly chopped
2 small apples, peeled and roughly chopped
6 cups Vegetable Stock (see page 272) or Chicken Stock (see page 272)
Freshly ground black pepper
A few chives, finely chopped, for serving

Heat the olive oil in a soup pot set over medium heat. Add the fennel, onion, and garlic along with a big pinch of salt and cook, stirring now and then, until softened but not browned, about 10 minutes.

Add the beets and apples to the pot and pour in the stock. Turn the heat to high, bring the soup to a boil, then turn the heat down and let the soup simmer until the beets and apples are completely soft, 30 to 35 minutes. Carefully puree the soup in a powerful blender and season to taste with salt and pepper. Serve with the chives sprinkled on top.

COLD AVOCADO + CUCUMBER SOUP

Really light and refreshing, this soup is also incredibly satisfying, since the avocado makes it so creamy. My grandmother used to make a soup like this that I loved as a kid.

Serves 4

E Elimination Diet **V** Vegan

Zest and juice of 3 limes
2 large cucumbers, peeled and seeded, roughly chopped
2 avocados, peeled and roughly chopped
1 teaspoon sea salt

Combine everything in a powerful blender and blitz until it's totally creamy and smooth.

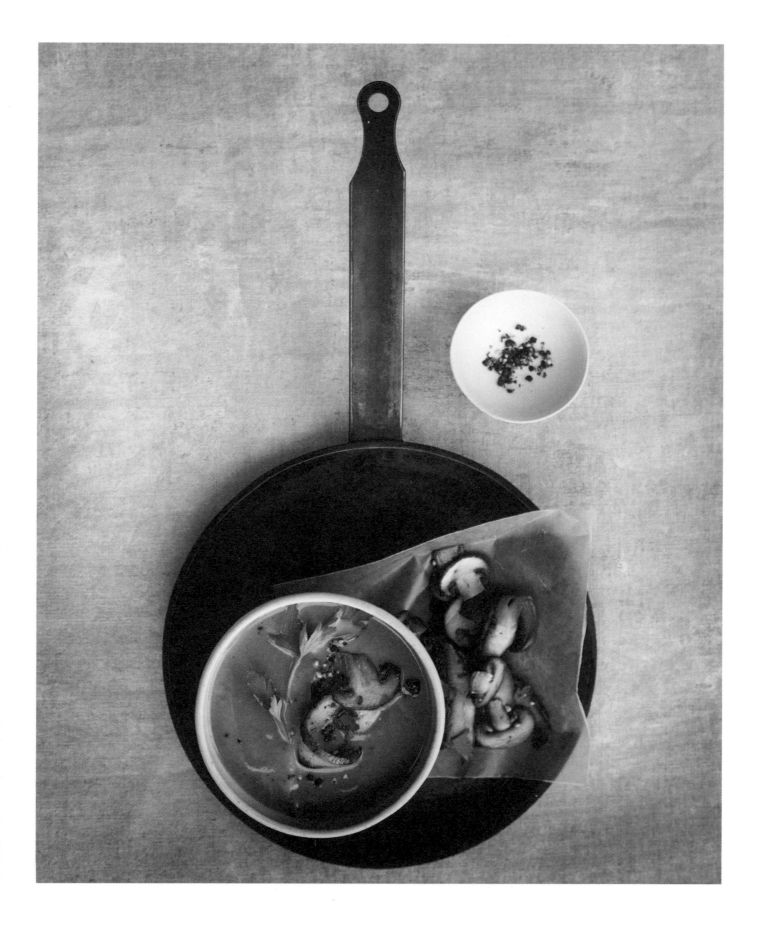

MANY-MUSHROOM SOUP

This soup gets so much depth of flavor from the dried mushrooms and such a creamy texture from being pureed that it's hard to believe no chicken stock or cream is involved. If you'd like to add a little texture, quickly sauté a few thin slices of the mushrooms in olive oil with some salt and pepper and float them in each bowl.

Serves about 6

E Elimination Diet **V** Vegan

3 dried shiitake mushrooms
½ cup boiling water
2 tablespoons extra virgin olive oil
3 leeks, white and light green parts only,
    thoroughly washed and finely chopped
1 small yellow onion, finely diced
2 garlic cloves, minced
1 teaspoon fresh thyme
Coarse sea salt
1 pound crimini mushrooms, stems removed and
    caps roughly chopped
1 large portobello mushroom, stem removed and
    cap roughly chopped
4 cups Vegetable Stock (see page 272)
Italian parsley for serving
Freshly ground black pepper

Place the shiitakes in a small bowl or teacup with the boiling water and set aside for at least 10 minutes. Drain the mushrooms, being sure to reserve their soaking liquid. Slice off and discard the stems and thinly slice the caps and set them aside.

Meanwhile, heat the olive oil in a large, heavy pot over medium-high heat. Add the leeks, onion, garlic, and thyme, along with 2 heavy pinches of salt, and cook, stirring now and then, until softened but not browned, 9 or 10 minutes. Add the crimini and portobello mushrooms and the reserved shiitake mushrooms. Stir to combine with the leek mixture and cook until the mushrooms begin to release their liquid, 5 to 6 minutes.

Add the vegetable stock and the reserved mushroom soaking liquid (avoid any grit that might be at the bottom) to the pot and turn up the heat. Once the soup comes to a boil, lower the heat and simmer for 20 minutes to bring it all together.

Carefully puree in a powerful blender. If you want a really refined, smooth texture, you can pass the pureed soup through a fine-mesh strainer. Serve immediately with a bit of parsley for color and a healthy grind of black pepper.

CHICKEN SOUP WITH KALE + CARROTS

This bubbles on my stove all winter long—practically Jewish penicillin. The men in my house love this soup.

Serves 4, with leftovers

E Elimination Diet **P** Protein-Packed

1 whole 3- to 4-pound organic chicken, washed
1 celery stalk, roughly chopped
1 large leek, thoroughly washed and roughly
    chopped (including the dark green part)
1 large carrot, peeled and roughly chopped, plus
    2 more carrots, peeled and diced
1 yellow onion, quartered
1 bay leaf
2 leafy sprigs of thyme
½ teaspoon whole black peppercorns
2 teaspoons coarse sea salt
1 bunch of kale, leaves stripped off the stems,
    in bite-sized pieces
Freshly ground black pepper

Combine the chicken, the celery, the leek, the 1 roughly chopped carrot, the onion, the bay leaf, the thyme, the peppercorns, and the salt in a large soup pot and cover with cold water (it will take about 10 cups). Bring the soup to a boil over high heat, then lower the heat and simmer the soup for 2 hours. Strain the stock into a clean soup pot and discard the cooked vegetables. Pull the white meat off the chicken and cut into a rough dice. Reserve the dark meat for another use (or you can add it to the soup if you like). Add the diced chicken breast, the 2 diced carrots, and the kale to the soup and simmer for an additional 20 minutes. Season to taste with salt and pepper.

WHITE BEAN + SWISS CHARD SOUP

This simple soup is enriched with lots of texture by simply pureeing some of the soup itself. A really satisfying vegetarian option, this combination of beans and greens gives you ample protein. Note that you can substitute any dark leafy green for the Swiss chard—mustard greens add a really lovely spicy kick.

Serves 4

E Elimination Diet **V** Vegan

2 tablespoons extra virgin olive oil
2 leeks, thoroughly washed and finely chopped
1 large yellow onion, finely diced
2 garlic cloves, minced
1 bay leaf
Coarse sea salt
4 cups Vegetable Stock (see page 272)
A 14-ounce can cannellini or gigante beans
1 bunch of Swiss chard, leaves roughly chopped
    and stems discarded
Freshly ground black pepper

Heat the olive oil in a large, heavy pot over medium heat. Add the leeks, onion, garlic, and bay leaf along with a heavy pinch of salt and cook, stirring now and then, until softened but not browned, 10 minutes.

Add the vegetable stock and the beans to the pot and turn up the heat. Once the soup comes to a boil, lower the heat and simmer until everything has completely softened and the soup is wonderfully fragrant, about 20 minutes. Remove and discard the bay leaf.

Carefully puree 2 cups of the soup in a powerful blender and return it to the pot. Add the Swiss chard leaves and cook over medium-high heat just until they've wilted, about 3 minutes. Season the soup with salt and pepper to taste and serve immediately.

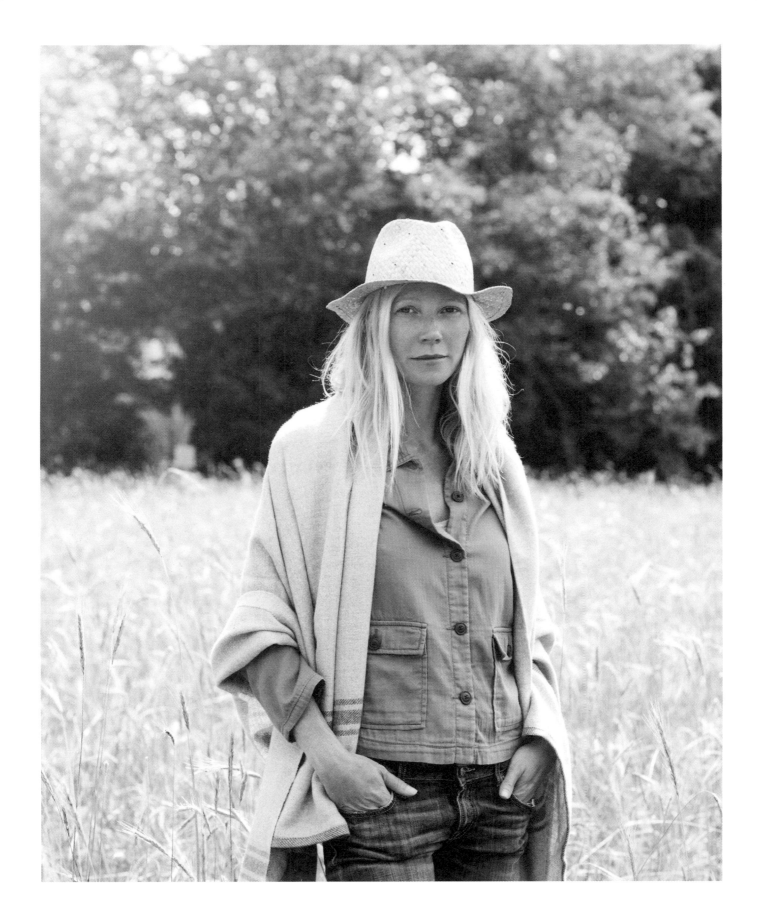

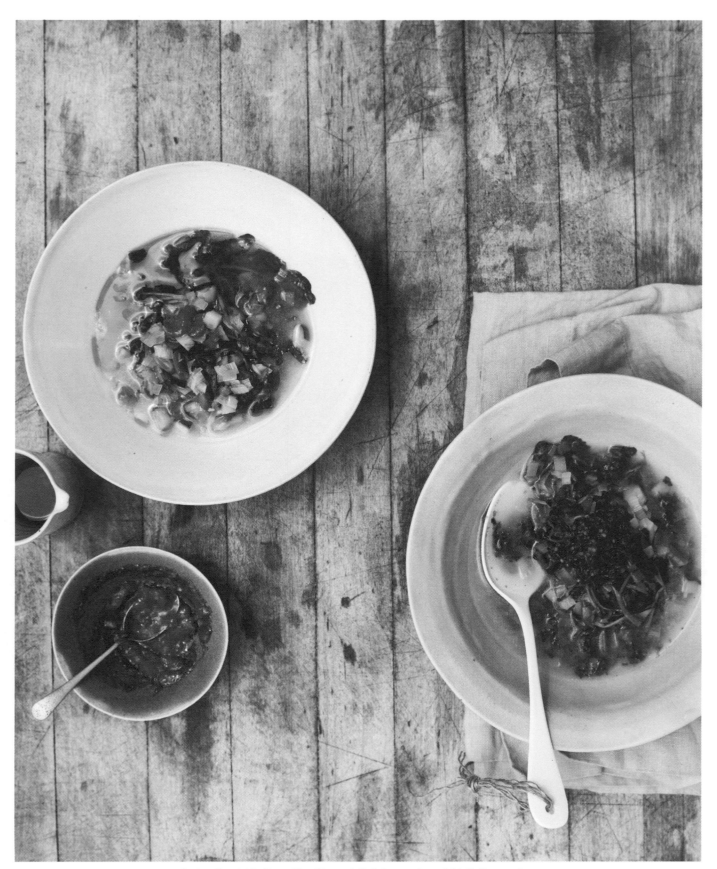

Spring Vegetable Soup, Two Ways—*left*, Asian version; *right*, Italian version

SPRING VEGETABLE SOUP, TWO WAYS

The base of this soup—sautéed leeks and garlic, good stock, and a lovely variety of spring vegetables—couldn't be easier to prepare. It's delicious on its own, but it can also quickly and easily be finished in two very different cultural directions: Asian, with a bit of soy sauce, sesame oil, and sriracha, or Italian, with a spoonful of pesto—try them both!

Serves 4

E Elimination Diet **V** Vegan

2 tablespoons extra virgin olive oil
2 large leeks, thoroughly washed and finely
    chopped
2 garlic cloves, finely minced
Coarse sea salt
4 cups Vegetable Stock (see page 272)
1 small zucchini, finely diced (about ⅔ cup)
A handful of haricots verts, cut into ¼-inch pieces
    (about ½ cup)
2 packed cups baby spinach or watercress
Soy sauce, toasted sesame oil, and Lee's Sriracha
    (see page 274) for the Asian version
A few spoonfuls of Classic Pesto (see page 285)
    for the Italian version

Heat the olive oil in a large, heavy pot over medium heat. Add the leeks and garlic, along with a heavy pinch of salt, and cook, stirring now and then, until softened but not browned, 10 minutes.

Add the vegetable stock and turn up the heat. Once the soup comes to a boil, lower the heat and simmer for 10 minutes, just to get the leek flavor nicely acquainted with the stock. Add the zucchini and the haricots verts and cook until just tender, about 2 minutes. Add the spinach or watercress and cook until wilted, not even a full minute.

For the Asian version, serve with bottles of soy sauce, toasted sesame oil, and Lee's Sriracha and encourage your guests to stir in a few drops of each to taste.

For the Italian version, serve each portion with a big spoonful of Classic Pesto to be stirred in.

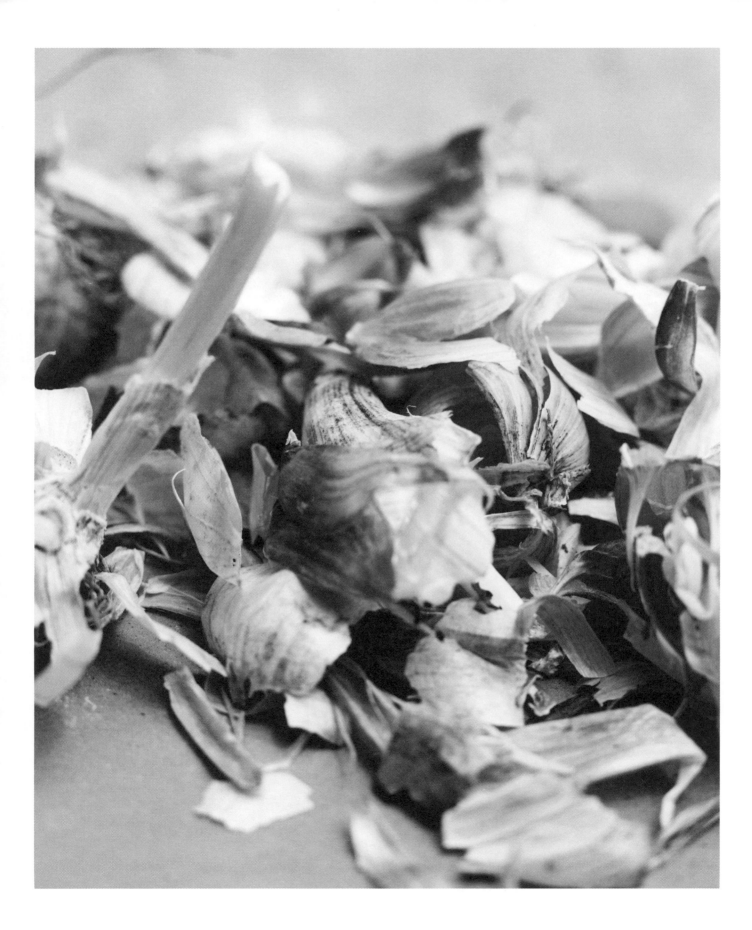

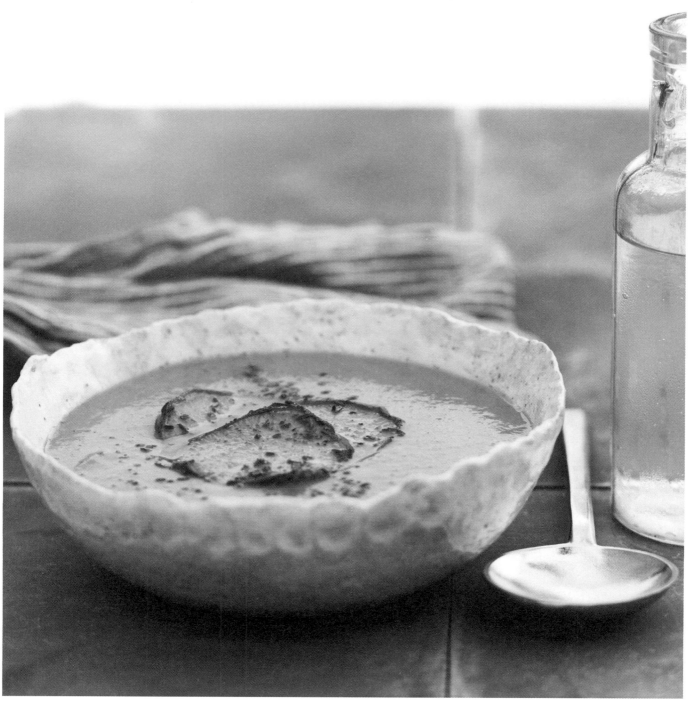

Spicy Sweet Potato Soup with Chipotle + Coriander (page 88)

SPICY SWEET POTATO SOUP WITH CHIPOTLE + CORIANDER

My gosh, this is the perfect soup…with its southwestern flavors and its creamy, rich texture without the dairy, you'll really feel as if you're having a treat. For a bit of extra texture, pan-fry a few pieces of sweet potato in a bit of olive oil with toasted ground cumin or coriander and slide them onto the finished soup before serving.

Serves 4

E Elimination Diet **V** Vegan

2 tablespoons extra virgin olive oil
1 large red onion, finely diced (about 1½ cups)
2 garlic cloves, minced
5 sprigs of cilantro, leaves reserved for garnish, stems tied together with a piece of kitchen string
¾ teaspoon cumin
Coarse sea salt
1½ teaspoons chipotle in adobo (or more if you like)
2 large sweet potatoes, peeled and diced (about 6 cups)
6 cups Vegetable Stock (see page 272)

Heat the olive oil in a large, heavy pot over medium heat. Add the onion, garlic, cilantro sprigs, cumin, and a heavy pinch of salt and cook, stirring now and then, until softened but not browned, 10 minutes. Add the chipotle and the sweet potatoes and stir to combine. Add the vegetable stock to the pot and turn up the heat. Once the soup comes to a boil, lower the heat and simmer until the sweet potatoes are very soft, about 30 minutes. Remove and discard the cilantro. Carefully puree the soup in a powerful blender. If you want a really refined, smooth texture, you can pass the pureed soup through a fine-mesh strainer. Garnish each bowl with a few of the reserved cilantro leaves.

BEET GREENS SOUP

This soup is all about the nutrient-dense, often-neglected, really tasty leaves attached to the tops of fresh beets. Since grocery stores and farmers' markets don't sell the leaves separate from the beets, you can either set the beets aside for another use (check out the Three Simple Beet Salads on page 155) or you can steam or roast them, peel them, and then finely slice them and slip them into the soup when you serve it.

Serves 4

E Elimination Diet
V Vegan (made with vegetable stock)

2 tablespoons extra virgin olive oil, plus more for
    serving
1 leek, washed well and diced
1 small fennel bulb, green parts discarded, white
    parts diced
1 yellow onion, diced
2 garlic cloves, finely minced
Greens from 1 bunch of beets, stems and leaves
    separated, washed and roughly chopped
Coarse sea salt
Freshly ground black pepper
6 cups Vegetable Stock (see page 272) or Chicken
    Stock (see page 272)

Heat the olive oil in a soup pot set over medium heat. Add the leek, fennel, onion, garlic, and beet stems and cook, stirring now and then, until softened, about 10 minutes. Try to avoid giving the vegetables color; just get them to sweat.

Add the beet greens to the vegetables along with a large pinch of salt and a few generous grinds of pepper. Stir to combine, then pour the stock over the vegetables. Turn the heat to high, bring the soup to a boil, and turn off the heat. You want the greens to be just wilted and still have their integrity. Carefully puree the soup in a powerful blender; if you'd like the texture to be extremely smooth, pass the soup through a fine-mesh strainer into a clean pot. Season to taste with more salt and pepper. This soup can be chilled and eaten cold. Serve with a drizzle of good olive oil and a grind of black pepper.

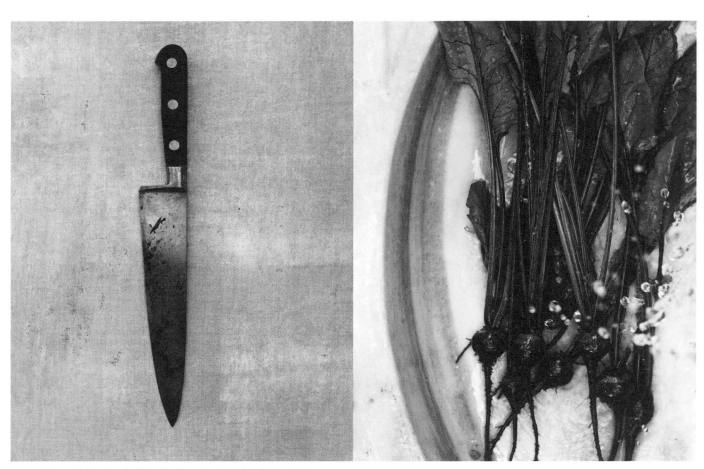

Bruce Paltrow's chef's knife, bought at E. Dehillerin, Paris,
and passed down to me.

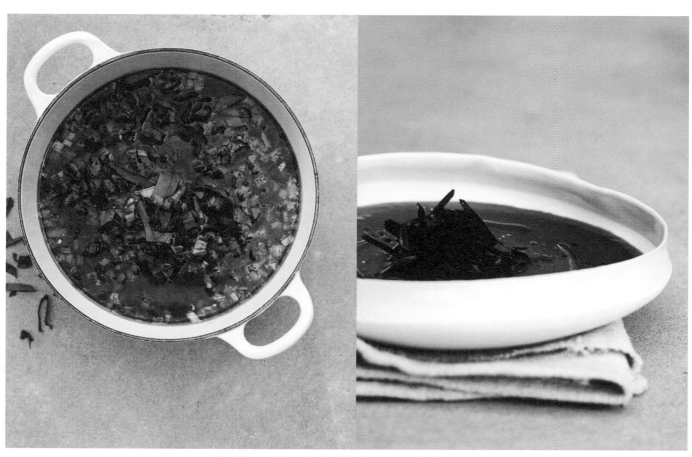

Beet Greens Soup—before blending, and after (page 89)

EASIEST POSOLE

Julia came up with this recipe on an unseasonably cold day one summer when I craved something warm and comforting that still had light, ever-so-spicy flavors. The various fresh vegetable garnishes allow everyone to customize their posole however they choose.

Serves 4

Ⓥ Vegan (made with vegetable stock)

FOR THE POSOLE
6 tomatilloes, papery layers and stems discarded, roughly chopped
1 large red onion, peeled and roughly chopped
2 jalapeños, roughly chopped (take out the seeds if you don't want it too spicy)
Extra virgin olive oil
Coarse sea salt
4 cups Vegetable Stock (see page 272) or Chicken Stock (see page 272)
3 large sprigs of cilantro
A 28-ounce can hominy, drained and rinsed

FOR THE GARNISH
1 ripe avocado, diced
A small handful of cilantro leaves
2 scallions, white and light green parts only, thinly sliced
2 or 3 radishes, thinly sliced
1 lime, cut into wedges

Preheat the oven to 450°F.

On a sheet pan or in a large baking dish, toss the tomatilloes, onions, and jalapeños with enough olive oil just to coat and a large pinch of salt. Roast, stirring now and then, until they're soft and a little browned, 20 minutes.

Transfer the roasted vegetables to a powerful blender along with 1 cup of the stock and puree until completely smooth (be very careful when blending hot ingredients). Transfer the mixture to a large pot along with the rest of the stock, the cilantro, and the hominy. Bring the mixture to a boil, lower the heat, and simmer for 15 minutes, or until all the flavors have completely gotten to know each other. Season the soup to taste with salt.

Remove the cilantro and serve the soup along with bowls of the avocado, cilantro leaves, scallions, radishes, and lime wedges and encourage your guests to add whatever they'd like to their posole.

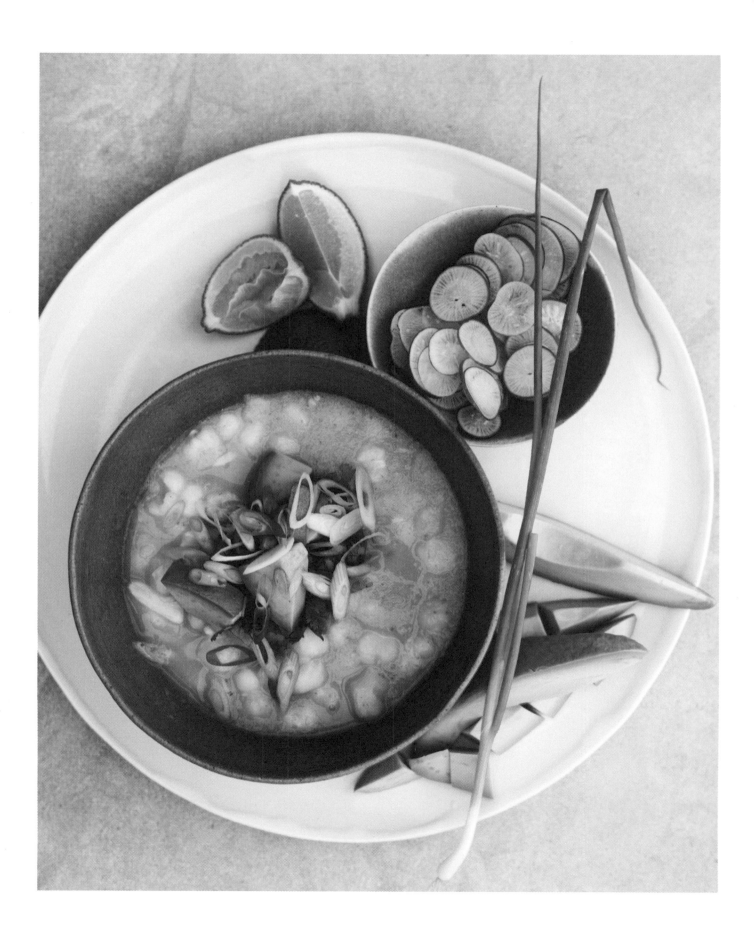

BIRDS + SOME MEAT

For a long time (after I read about factory farming) I didn't eat birds or meat. I am a firm believer in raising animals right and eating only organic, heritage, grass-fed, free-range ones—or even better, game birds from the wild, the way it was meant to be. Eating wild game birds is more expensive, but they taste better, and they're much better for you. In this chapter, Julia and I focus a lot on chicken, a lean, light protein that works with any diet (except a vegetarian or vegan one!). We have devised preparations that make chicken exciting again. We've also included a few other types of meat dishes for the carnivorous who are looking for leaner cuts but still want all the flavor.

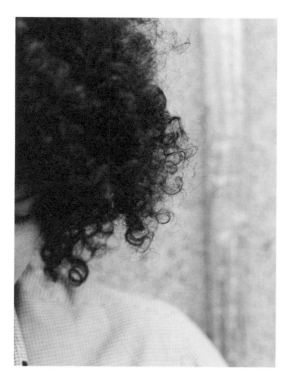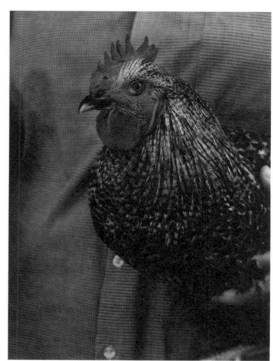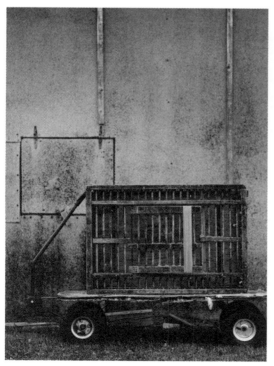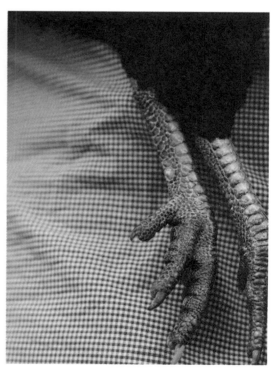

TERIYAKI CHICKEN

I first devised this recipe for GOOP.com when we were searching for a detox-friendly chicken recipe that had some real flavor. It's also very low in fat, if you're counting calories.

Serves 4

Ⓔ Elimination Diet Ⓟ Protein-Packed

FOR THE DETOX TERIYAKI SAUCE
⅓ cup balsamic vinegar
⅓ cup brown rice syrup or raw honey
1 teaspoon freshly grated ginger
¼ teaspoon freshly ground black pepper
1 teaspoon barley miso
1 teaspoon mirin
1 tablespoon water

FOR THE CHICKEN
4 chicken breasts
Detox Teriyaki Sauce
3 scallions, white and light green parts only, thinly sliced
A dozen sprigs of cilantro, roughly chopped

Combine the balsamic vinegar, syrup or honey, ginger, and pepper in a small saucepan. Bring to a boil, lower to a simmer, and cook for 10 minutes. Add the miso, mirin, and water and let cool.

Marinate the chicken in half of the sauce (reserve the rest) for at least 1 hour and as long as overnight.

Heat a grill or grill pan over medium heat. Wipe off any excess marinade and grill the chicken for 3 to 4 minutes on a side, or until cooked through. Serve with the reserved sauce, and the scallions and cilantro.

BARBECUED CHICKEN, SPANISH STYLE

The spice paste in this recipe allows the flavor to really get into the bird—the best bite is that line of spice between the meat and the skin. Don't be tempted to blast the chicken over high heat; grill it low and slow to let the fat work for it—the fat will render and keep the meat from drying out. If you want a bit more kick, it's nice to brush the chicken just at the end with adobo sauce (that great stuff that chipotles come packed in).

Serves 4

Ⓔ Elimination Diet Ⓟ Protein-Packed

¼ cup extra virgin olive oil
4 garlic cloves, finely minced
A large pinch of coarse sea salt
1 teaspoon freshly ground black pepper
2 teaspoons hot pimentón
2 teaspoons red wine vinegar
One 3- to 4-pound chicken, cut into pieces on
        the bone (2 legs, 2 thighs, both wings split
        at the joint, and you can cut each breast in
        half if you like)

Mix everything but the chicken in a small bowl. Rub the paste all over the chicken pieces, being sure to get plenty underneath the skin, too. If possible, set the chicken in the refrigerator and let it sit overnight. Take it out of the refrigerator 1 or 2 hours before cooking so it's not ice cold.

When you're ready to eat, heat a grill or grill pan over low heat. Cook the chicken for 20 minutes on a side (the legs and thighs might want 5 or 10 more minutes), or until it's firm to the touch and nicely browned and the skin is quite crispy.

BRAISED CHICKEN WITH GREEN OLIVES + LEMON

This is one of those recipes that is such rich comfort food, you won't realize you're cutting anything out. We cooked this using a half chicken so the bird could lie nice and flat in the pot. But you can easily double the recipe and use a whole bird; just brown it in batches…or get a bigger pot.

Serves 2

E Elimination Diet **P** Protein-Packed

½ chicken, cut up, at room temperature
Coarse sea salt
Freshly ground black pepper
2 tablespoons extra virgin olive oil
3 shallots, sliced into thin rings
1½ cups Chicken Stock (see page 272)
2 garlic cloves, peeled and cut in half
10 large green olives, pitted
Leaves from 1 sprig of thyme
Juice of 1 lemon

Generously salt and pepper the chicken on both sides.

Place the olive oil in a large enameled cast-iron pot (like a Le Creuset Dutch oven) set over high heat. Add the chicken, skin side down, and cook until deeply browned, 4 to 5 minutes. Turn the chicken over and let it brown on the second side, another 4 to 5 minutes. Remove the chicken to a plate and set aside.

Turn the heat to medium and add the shallots to the pot. Cook, stirring often, until they begin to soften, 3 to 4 minutes. Add a splash of the chicken stock and use a wooden spoon to loosen any bits of shallot or chicken that might be caught at the bottom of the pot (aka the best bits). Add the remaining stock to the pot and add the chicken, skin side up, along with any juice that's accumulated on the plate. Scatter the garlic cloves, olives, and thyme sprigs over the chicken. Evenly pour the lemon juice over all. Bring the mixture to a boil, turn the heat as low as it will go, cover the pot, and cook for 1 hour, or until the chicken is nearly falling off the bone.

Uncover the pot and raise the heat. Let the pot boil to reduce and thicken the sauce until it's the texture of a great gravy—not too thin, not too thick—5 to 6 minutes. Serve hot with something that will sop up all of the lovely juice (any cooked grain, including polenta, would be really nice).

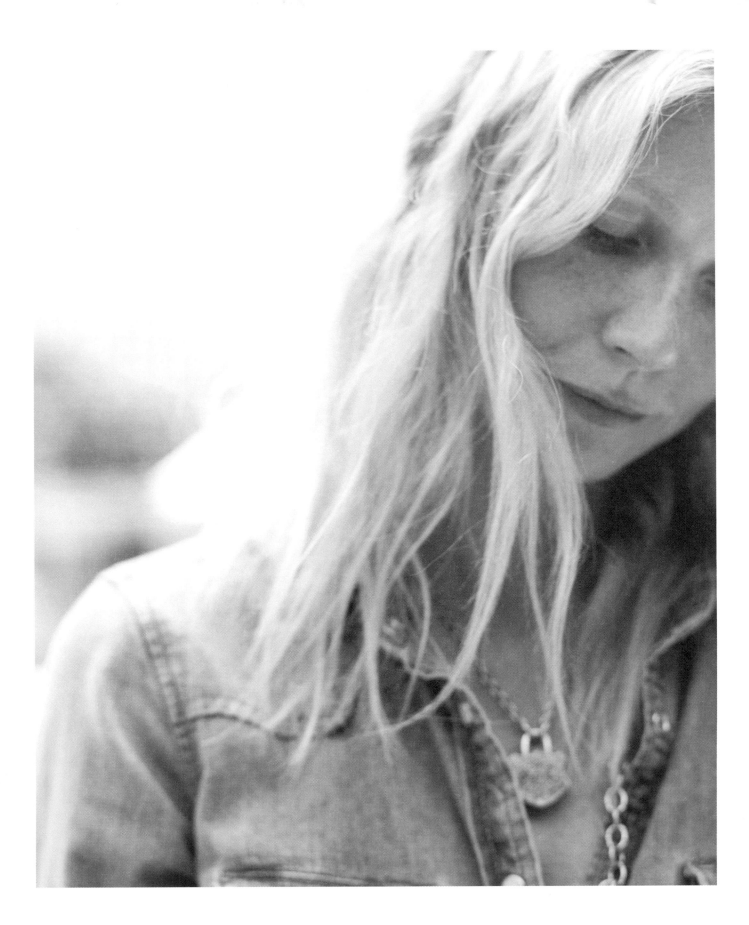

PERFECT HERBED GRILLED CHICKEN

This is a beautifully simple, very-low-fat chicken recipe that isn't boring, and it's ready in no time. The fresh herb rub really takes everyday grilled chicken to another level.

Serves 4

E Elimination Diet **P** Protein-Packed

1 teaspoon very, very finely chopped fresh sage
1 teaspoon very, very finely chopped fresh thyme
1 teaspoon very, very finely chopped fresh
    rosemary
1 tablespoon very, very finely chopped fresh
    Italian parsley
1 tablespoon very, very finely chopped fresh basil
1 small garlic clove, finely minced
¼ cup extra virgin olive oil
Zest of ½ lemon
2 tablespoons freshly squeezed lemon juice
½ teaspoon coarse sea salt
4 boneless, skinless chicken breasts pounded to
    barely ¼ inch thick

Combine the herbs, garlic, olive oil, lemon zest, lemon juice, and salt in a large mixing bowl. Add the chicken breasts to the bowl and rub the herb mixture all over each piece, being sure to get it on both sides. Cover the bowl with plastic wrap and let the chicken marinate for at least ½ hour, or as long as overnight.

Heat a grill or grill pan over medium heat. Grill the chicken until just cooked through, about 2 minutes on each side.

SUPER-CRISPY ROAST CHICKEN

This dish is in heavy rotation at my home—the men in my house *love* it. The recipe is totally simple and perfect; serve it with White Bean Puree with Turnip + Roasted Garlic (see page 163) and a green veggie and you have an ultrahealthy comfort food dinner.

Serves 4

E Elimination Diet **P** Protein-Packed

A high-quality 4-pound chicken
Coarse sea salt
Freshly ground black pepper
2 tablespoons extra virgin olive oil
½ lemon
½ small yellow onion, peeled

Preheat the oven to 425°F

Wash and thoroughly dry the chicken. Sprinkle a generous amount of salt and pepper inside the cavity, then rub the entire bird with olive oil. Sprinkle salt and pepper on the underside of the chicken and place it, breast side up, in a roasting dish. Stuff the cavity with the lemon and onion and generously sprinkle the top with salt and pepper.

Roast the chicken for 1½ hours, basting every ½ hour with the juices that accumulate in the pan. The chicken thigh should register 165°F on a digital thermometer at the very least (I usually let it get to 180°F just to be completely sure it's cooked all the way through the bone). Let the chicken rest for at least 10 minutes before carving and eating. After removing the chicken from the oven, be sure to pour about ½ cup of boiling water into the roasting dish; use a wooden spoon to scrape up all the browned bits from the bottom of the pan and serve the chicken with these rich pan juices.

CHICKEN FRANCESE

Yum. Italian comfort food done in a gluten-free style.

Serves 4

Ⓟ Protein-Packed

4 boneless, skinless chicken breasts
Coarse sea salt
Freshly ground black pepper
2 cups gluten-free flour
3 large eggs
Extra virgin olive oil
2 tablespoons finely chopped Italian parsley
1 lemon, cut into wedges

Using a mallet, pound the chicken breasts until they're about ¼ inch thick. Season both sides of each piece of chicken with a pinch of salt and pepper. Place the flour on a plate and lightly dust both sides of each piece of chicken with the flour. Beat the eggs in a shallow bowl with a big pinch of salt and a few grinds of pepper and set aside.

Heat ¼ cup of olive oil over medium-high heat in a nonstick skillet big enough to hold 2 pieces of the chicken in a single layer. Dip 2 pieces of the floured chicken into the egg mixture and coat on both sides, holding them up over the bowl for a second to drain any excess. Carefully place both pieces of floured-and-egged chicken in the skillet and cook about 4 minutes on the first side, or until evenly browned and crisp. Flip and cook for an additional 2 or 3 minutes, or until the other side is browned and crisp and the chicken is firm to the touch. Place the cooked chicken on a warm platter, wipe out the skillet, and repeat the process with ¼ cup fresh olive oil, the remaining 2 pieces of chicken, and the remaining flour and beaten egg. Serve the chicken sprinkled with parsley and drizzled with a healthy amount of fresh lemon juice.

CHICKEN + WHITE BEAN CHILI

I usually have a pot of chili on the stove all winter, as my daughter loves the veggie kind and asks for it all the time. This one boosts the protein quotient with chicken breasts.

Serves 4

Ⓟ Protein-Packed

3 chicken breasts on the bone with their skin (or 1 whole 3- to 4-pound chicken, cut up), at room temperature
3 tablespoons extra virgin olive oil, divided
Coarse sea salt
Freshly ground black pepper
2 small yellow onions, diced (about 2 cups)
1 red bell pepper, seeds and stem discarded, diced (about 1 cup)
3 garlic cloves, minced
¾ teaspoon ground cumin
½ teaspoon chili powder
½ teaspoon sweet pimentón
A 28-ounce can whole peeled tomatoes with their juice
A 14-ounce can cannellini or navy beans, rinsed and drained
Toppings (choose 1 or more): cilantro, lime wedges, finely diced red onion, hot sauce, plain sheep's or goat's milk yogurt

Preheat the oven to 425°F. Rub the chicken breasts or cut-up pieces with 1 tablespoon of olive oil, season aggressively with salt and pepper, and set them on a parchment-lined sheet pan. Roast until they're very firm to the touch and just cooked through, about 25 minutes. Once the chicken is cool enough to handle, remove the skin and bones and shred the meat with your fingers. Set it aside.

Meanwhile, heat the remaining 2 tablespoons of olive oil in a large soup pot set over medium-high heat. Add the onions, bell pepper, garlic, cumin, chili powder, pimentón, and a large pinch of salt. Cook, stirring now and then, until the vegetables are softened but not browned, about 10 minutes. Add the tomatoes and another pinch of salt and turn the heat up. Once the mixture comes to a boil, turn the heat to low and cook for ½ hour, or until the tomatoes begin to break down and lose their tinny taste. Break the tomatoes up a bit with the back of your spoon and add the beans and the reserved chicken to the pot, stirring to combine. Add a splash of water (about ⅓ cup) if the chili is looking a bit dry and simmer for another 15 to 20 minutes before seasoning to taste with salt and pepper. Serve with whatever toppings you like.

MR. CHOW—STYLE MINCED CHICKEN WITH LETTUCE LEAVES

I love a lettuce wrap. While trying to dream up ways of making low-fat, low-carb, preservative-free yet utterly happy food, I remembered venerable Mr. Chow's Squab with Lettuce. We devised this very tasty, very healthy version, which is great as a passed hors d'oeuvre or as a first course. This can also be made vegetarian by leaving out the chicken and adding a cup of chopped water chestnuts to the vegetable mixture.

Serves 4

(P) Protein-Packed

Neutral oil (like canola, grapeseed, or
    safflower oil)
1 pound ground chicken (preferably dark meat),
    at room temperature
Coarse sea salt
Freshly ground black pepper
1 yellow onion, peeled and finely diced
4 garlic cloves, finely minced
2 tablespoons finely minced fresh ginger
2 small carrots or 1 large carrot, peeled and finely
    diced (about ½ cup)
½ cup finely diced lotus root (optional)
1 recipe of Lee's Hoisin Sauce (page 275), divided
1 head of Bibb or iceberg lettuce, leaves
    separated
A handful of cilantro leaves
A few scallions, white and light green parts only,
    thinly sliced
Lee's Sriracha (see page 274), for serving

Heat a few tablespoonfuls of oil in a large, heavy skillet set over medium-high heat and add the chicken, along with a healthy pinch of salt and a few grinds of black pepper. Cook, stirring now and then to break the chicken up, until its liquid has been released and has evaporated and the meat is nicely browned, a good 10 to15 minutes.

Meanwhile, heat another couple of spoonfuls of oil in a separate skillet over medium-high heat and add the onion, garlic, and ginger. Cook, stirring now and then, until the mixture is just beginning to soften, about 5 minutes. Add the carrot, the lotus root if you're using it, and a big pinch of salt and cook until the carrot just begins to soften, about 10 minutes. Combine the chicken and the vegetables in 1 pan and add ½ cup of Lee's Hoisin Sauce along with ½ cup of water; cook for a final minute or 2 to just bring everything together. Place spoonfuls of the mixture on the lettuce leaves until you've used it all up (this recipe makes about a dozen wraps, but it depends how big your lettuce leaves are!). Thin the remainder of the Lee's Hoisin Sauce with ½ cup of water and drizzle a bit on top of each lettuce cup. Scatter the cilantro and scallions over the lettuce cups and serve with Lee's Sriracha if anyone wants a little kick.

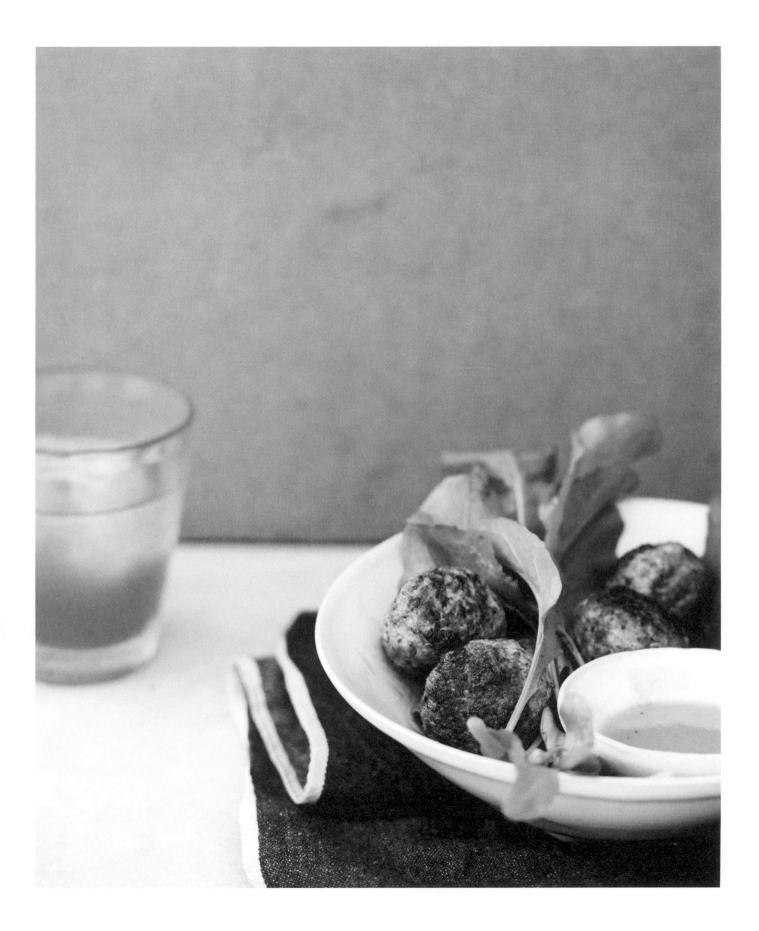

TURKEY MEATBALLS

No food makes me feel more comforted than spaghetti and meatballs, and that's always been the way. I have moved from pork and veal to the turkey variety in an ongoing effort to clean up my diet, but my meatballs still have dairy (cheese), gluten (bread crumbs), and egg. One afternoon, we devised this incredibly easy, incredibly good "friendly" version that still does the trick.

Serves 4 (makes 2 dozen golf ball–sized meatballs)

(E) Elimination Diet (make without the tomato sauce and simply cook the meatballs in the pan the whole way through, or bake them)
(P) Protein-Packed

1 small onion, roughly chopped
2 garlic cloves, roughly chopped
8 fresh sage leaves
8 large fresh basil leaves
Leaves from 4 sprigs of thyme
Leaves from a 5-inch sprig of rosemary
¼ cup Italian parsley
1 large handful of arugula roughly chopped
1 pound ground turkey
1 teaspoon coarse sea salt
½ teaspoon freshly ground black pepper
4 cups (1 recipe) Go-To Tomato Sauce
    (see page 273)
3 tablespoons extra virgin olive oil

Combine the onion, garlic, herbs, and arugula in the bowl of a food processor and pulse until very finely chopped. Transfer the mixture to a large mixing bowl along with the turkey, salt, and pepper. Use your hands to thoroughly combine all the ingredients, then roll the mixture into golf ball–sized meatballs.

Place the Go-To Tomato Sauce in a large pot set over low heat and let it get warm.

While the sauce is warming, heat the olive oil in a large nonstick skillet over medium-high heat. Cook the meatballs, in batches if necessary, until they're browned all over, 2 to 3 minutes on a side. Transfer the browned meatballs to the simmering tomato sauce and partially cover the pot. Let the meatballs cook gently for ½ hour, carefully stirring every now and then to make sure they're cooking evenly. Serve hot with your favorite gluten-free pasta, a pot of polenta, or even on their own alongside some Broccoli Rabe (see page 154).

TURKEY + BLACK BEAN CHILI WITH SWEET POTATOES

I love this protein-packed, delicious chili, which can be made vegan by substituting another can of black beans for the turkey. You can also add a spoonful of chipotle along with the tomatoes if you want more spice.

Serves 4

ⓟ Protein-Packed

2 sweet potatoes, peeled and cut into
    ¾-inch pieces
¼ cup extra virgin olive oil, divided
Coarse sea salt
1 large yellow onion, diced (about 1½ cups)
2 garlic cloves, minced
1 teaspoon ground cumin
½ teaspoon sweet pimentón
½ teaspoon mild chili powder
1 pound ground turkey (preferably dark meat)
A 28-ounce can whole peeled tomatoes
A 14-ounce can black beans, rinsed and drained
Chopped fresh cilantro and scallions for serving,
    if desired
Pickled Jalapeños (see page 280) and Spicy
    Cashew Moment (see page 286) for serving,
    if desired

Preheat the oven to 400°F.

Toss the sweet potatoes with 2 tablespoons of the olive oil and spread them out on a parchment-lined baking sheet. Evenly sprinkle with a good pinch of salt and roast, stirring now and then, until soft, about 20 minutes. Set aside.

Meanwhile, heat the remaining 2 tablespoons of olive oil in a large heavy-bottomed pot set over medium heat. Add the onion, garlic, cumin, pimentón, chili powder, and a big pinch of salt and cook, stirring now and then, until nice and soft but not too browned, 8 to 10 minutes. Add the turkey to the pan and cook, stirring now and then to break it up, until its liquid has been released and has evaporated and the meat is nicely browned. This will take a good 20 minutes, and it's worth being patient (don't be tempted to turn the heat up just to get a char on the turkey; the slow browning allows all the onion and spice flavor to really get in there).

Add the tomatoes and a large pinch of salt to the pot and turn the heat to high. Swish ½ cup of water in the tomato can to get all the tomato bits off and add this liquid to the pot, too. Once the mixture comes to a boil, turn the heat to low and let the chili simmer for 20 minutes. Use the back of your wooden spoon to crush the tomatoes as they cook.

Add the beans and the reserved sweet potatoes to the chili and continue to simmer for another 15 minutes, just to let it all come together. Serve with a scattering of cilantro and scallions, a few Pickled Jalapeños, and a dollop of Spicy Cashew Moment if you like.

TANDOORI TURKEY KABOBS

Turkey, an ideal lean meat, is a versatile protein to build a meal around. The tasty marinade makes this preparation full of flavor.

Serves 4

Ⓟ Protein-Packed

½ cup plain sheep's or goat's milk yogurt
½ teaspoon finely minced fresh ginger
½ teaspoon ground coriander
½ teaspoon ground cumin
½ teaspoon ground turmeric
A pinch of cayenne pepper
½ teaspoon coarse sea salt
1 lime
1 pound boneless, skinless turkey breast, cut into
    1-inch cubes
2 tablespoons roughly chopped cilantro

Soak a dozen 6-inch wooden skewers in water.

Whisk together the yogurt, spices, and salt. Zest the lime and add the zest to the yogurt mixture. Hold on to that lime—you'll need it later. Add the turkey to the yogurt mixture, mix to combine, and cover with a piece of plastic wrap. Marinate in the refrigerator for at least 1 hour and as long as overnight.

When you're ready to eat, heat a grill or grill pan over medium-high heat. Drain the skewers and thread the turkey on them (each skewer should get 4 or 5 pieces of turkey).

Brush the grill or grill pan with oil and grill the kabobs until firm to the touch and completely cooked through, about 3 minutes on a side.

Remove the kabobs to a platter. Cut your zested lime in half and squeeze the juice over the kabobs. Scatter cilantro over them and serve.

MIDDLE EASTERN TURKEY BURGERS WITH CUCUMBER + YOGURT SAUCE

Peppering turkey burgers with herbs and greens and serving them with a cooling yogurt sauce studded with crunchy cucumber makes for an unexpected, satisfying lunch. These are especially good alongside NY Street Vendor Salad (see page 62) or Roasted Eggplant with Tahini Dressing, Date Molasses + Mint (see page 166).

Makes 4 burgers

E Elimination Diet (skip the sauce) **P** Protein-Packed

4 shallots, roughly chopped (about ½ cup)
2 small cloves garlic, crushed
2 teaspoons dried oregano crushed with your
     fingertips
8 large basil leaves
3 handfuls baby spinach
Zest of 1 lemon
1 teaspoon coarse sea salt
½ teaspoon freshly ground black pepper
1 pound ground turkey (preferably dark meat)
2 tablespoons extra virgin olive oil

Blitz the shallots, garlic, oregano, basil, spinach, lemon zest, salt, and pepper together in a food processor until finely chopped. Place the mixture in a large bowl along with the turkey and mix with your hands or a rubber spatula to thoroughly combine. Form the mixture into 4 patties. At this point it's ideal to refrigerate the burgers for at least 1 hour and as long as overnight, to really let the flavors settle in, but they'll still be A-OK if you don't have this extra time.

Heat a grill or grill pan over medium-high heat. Brush the burgers with the olive oil and cook until firm to the touch and nicely browned, 7 to 8 minutes per side. Serve with the yogurt sauce.

YOGURT SAUCE

Makes about 1½ cups

1 cup plain sheep's milk or goat's milk yogurt
½ English cucumber, peeled and finely diced
     (about ½ cup)
2 scallions, white and light green parts only,
     thinly sliced
Leaves from 2 sprigs of mint, finely sliced
1 tablespoon finely chopped chives
½ teaspoon coarse sea salt

Mix all the ingredients in a bowl until blended.

BEST ROASTED TURKEY BREAST

This turkey is so good to have around—my family and I especially love it sliced for club sandwich lettuce wraps, the best go-to, no-carb, high-protein snack. For deli love without the gnarly processed deli turkey or the put-you-to-sleep kaiser roll, take a big piece of lettuce, thinly slice a bit of the roasted turkey, and wrap it up with a bit of Vegenaise and a slice of cooked turkey bacon. Or swap the turkey bacon for some sauerkraut and mix a little ketchup with the Vegenaise and voilà, a healthy Reuben! Get a Bubbies pickle and call it a day.

Serves 6 to 8

Ⓟ Protein-Packed

1 whole, organic boneless turkey breast
    (about 3 pounds)
Coarse sea salt
A 12-ounce bottle good-quality maple syrup
1 tablespoon extra virgin olive oil
Freshly ground black pepper

Place the turkey breast in a large bowl or pot that leaves tons of room around and on top of it. Sprinkle the turkey with a handful of salt—a good ¼ cup. Pour the maple syrup over the turkey and fill the bowl or pot with enough cold water to cover the turkey. Wrap the bowl or pot with plastic wrap and park it in the fridge overnight.

Take the turkey out of the fridge at least 1 hour before you're ready to roast it, to get it to room temperature. Pour off the brine. Preheat your oven to 425°F (preferably on convection, if that's possible).

Place the turkey, skin side up, in a roasting pan, patting it dry with paper towels. Rub the turkey with the olive oil and give it a tiny sprinkle of coarse salt (it doesn't need much, since it's been brined) and a few grinds of black pepper.

Roast for 15 minutes, turn the oven down to 375°F, and continue to roast until the turkey reaches 180°F on a meat thermometer (while 165°F is usually advised for poultry, we like it quite well done—to each his or her own; just don't take it out before it hits 165°F). The time will depend on how big a piece of meat you've got on your hands, but 45 minutes is average. Start taking the temperature after 25 minutes to be sure. Once it's cooked, let the turkey rest on a cutting board at least 15 minutes before slicing it.

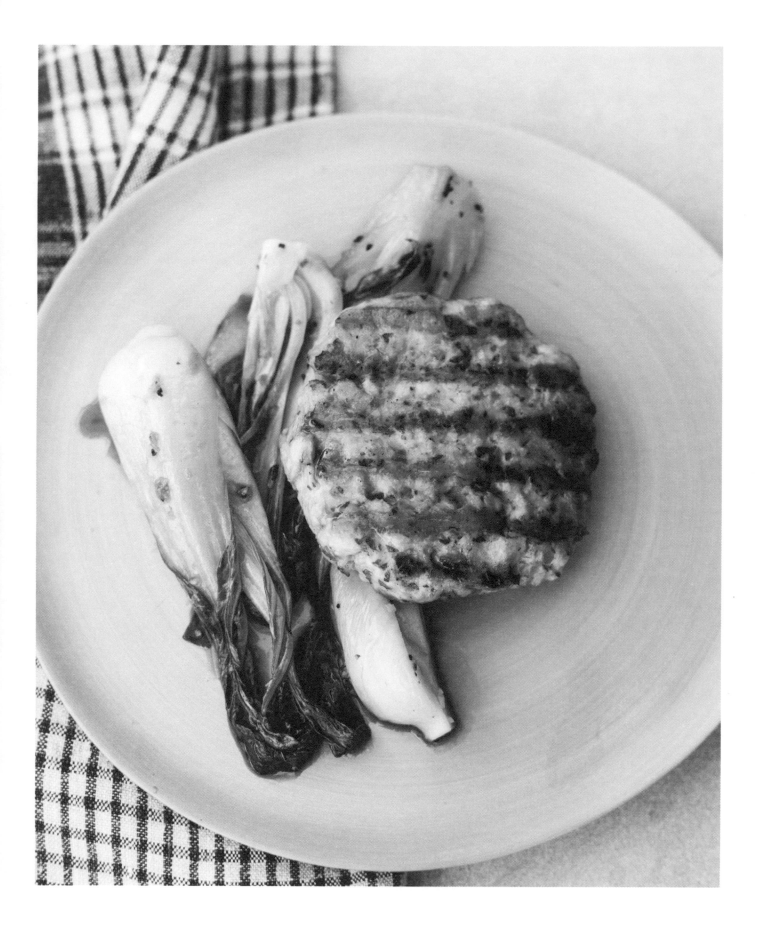

CHICKEN BURGERS, THAI STYLE

These were invented when I was trying to think up new and flavorful ways to use chicken while keeping out bad stuff. Insanely flavorful, these can be served with a side salad or on a gluten-free bun.

Serves 4

E Elimination Diet **P** Protein-Packed

1 pound ground chicken (preferably dark meat)
2 garlic cloves, very finely minced
⅔ cup cilantro, finely chopped
2 shallots, very finely minced
1 teaspoon very finely minced red chili (or more
    or less, however hot you like it)
2 teaspoons fish sauce
½ teaspoon coarse sea salt
½ teaspoon freshly ground black pepper
2 tablespoons neutral oil (like canola, grapeseed,
    or safflower oil)

Thoroughly mix the chicken with the garlic, cilantro, shallots, red chili, fish sauce, salt, and pepper. Form the mixture into 4 burgers, each about ¾ inch thick.

Heat a grill or grill pan over medium heat. Rub each burger on both sides with a bit of the safflower oil and grill for about 8 minutes on the first side and another 5 minutes on the second, or until nicely marked and firm to the touch.

TWO-PAN CHICKEN WITH HARISSA, PRESERVED LEMONS + GREEN OLIVES

Julia here. Gwyneth first started making this at home in London, and I will never forget the day when I first saw her lift the top pan off to reveal the crispiest roast chicken I'd ever seen. She had marinated it in garlic, lemon, and herbs, and we threw together some Salsa Verde (see page 284), and I thought dinner, not to mention life in general, couldn't really get much better. As we continued to tweak the technique, we started playing around with the flavors, too, and landed on this North African variation—it's pretty sensational. We also sometimes do a Korean version, switching the harissa to a paste made of gochujang (Korean red pepper paste, available at Asian markets and Hmart.com), mashed garlic and ginger, soy sauce, and a drop of sesame oil. If you go for that, be sure to serve it alongside Korean Slaw (see page 161) and Grilled Corn, Korean Style (see page 158). No matter which variation you choose—even if it's just salt and pepper—this chicken never disappoints. Note that you'll need a deboned chicken (your butcher can help you out) and two cast-iron pans—a large one big enough to hold the chicken laid out flat and one either the same size or just slightly smaller to sit right on top.

Serves 4

Ⓟ Protein-Packed

¼ cup harissa paste
Extra virgin olive oil
Coarse sea salt
1 deboned 3- to 4-pound chicken with the skin
     intact (your butcher can do this for you)
1 preserved lemon, roughly sliced
A small handful of pitted green olives, roughly
     chopped (about ⅔ cup)
2 teaspoons fresh oregano, finely chopped
Freshly ground black pepper
2 tablespoons high-quality raw honey, if desired

In a small bowl, mix together the harissa with ¼ cup olive oil and 1 teaspoon salt. Place the chicken in a baking dish or a large, shallow bowl—something that it can rest flat in. Use your fingers to gently make space between the chicken skin and the meat (including the legs). Rub half the harissa mixture underneath the skin on the entire bird. Do your best not to tear the skin (though if it happens, it's not the end of the world). Rub the rest of the paste all over both sides of the chicken. Be careful not to touch your face or eyes with the harissa on your hands.

Cover the dish with plastic wrap and set the chicken in the fridge for a few hours, preferably overnight—and if you're really planning ahead, as long as 2 days.

When you're ready to cook, take the chicken out of the fridge and let it come to room temperature. Meanwhile, preheat the oven to 500°F and park one cast-iron pan (the smaller one if you have different sizes) in the oven to get hot. Set the larger pan over high heat on the stovetop and hit it with a few glugs of olive oil (about ¼ cup). Carefully place the chicken, skin side down, in the hot pan. Let the chicken cook until the skin begins to brown, about 5 minutes. Carefully take the hot pan out of the oven and brush the bottom of it with a spoonful of olive oil, or spray it with cooking spray if you've got that on hand. Set the hot oiled skillet on top of the chicken. Very carefully set the whole thing in the oven and roast for exactly 20 minutes.

Meanwhile, combine the preserved lemon with the olives and oregano in a small bowl. Stir in a hit of extra virgin olive oil (about 2 tablespoons), a large pinch of coarse salt, and a few grinds of pepper. Set the mixture aside while the chicken is in the oven.

After 20 minutes, very carefully remove the chicken and its pans from the oven. Set the top pan aside, remove the chicken to a board, and let it sit for 5 to 10 minutes to let the juices evenly distribute themselves, which will make the chicken easier to cut up. After it's rested, cut the chicken into pieces and serve immediately, topped with the preserved lemon mixture. If you'd like a sweet note, serve it with a little raw honey, too.

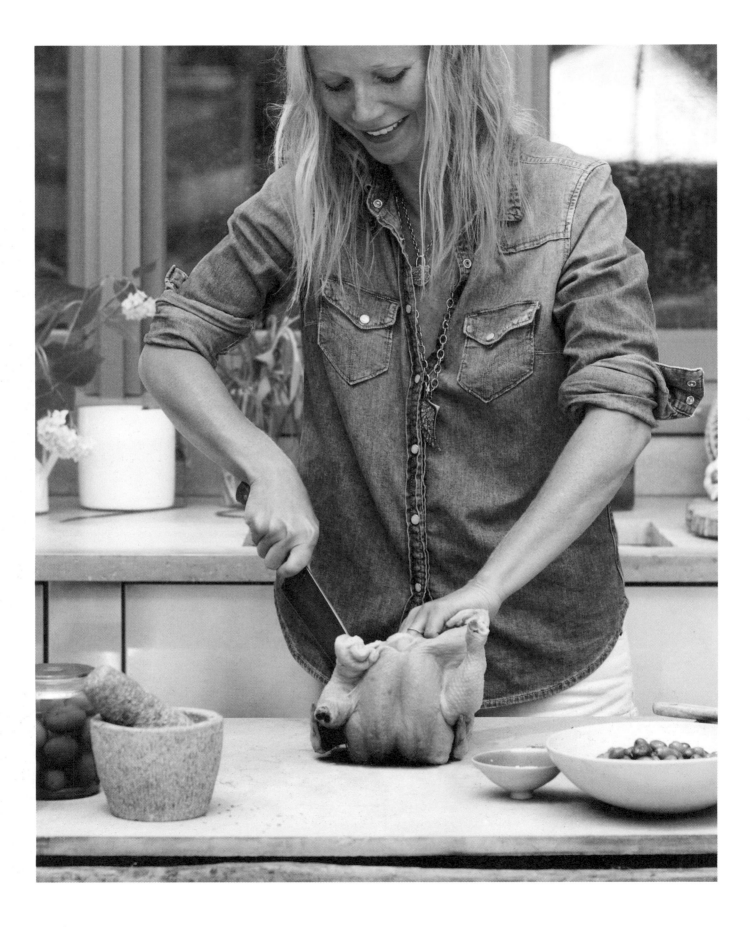

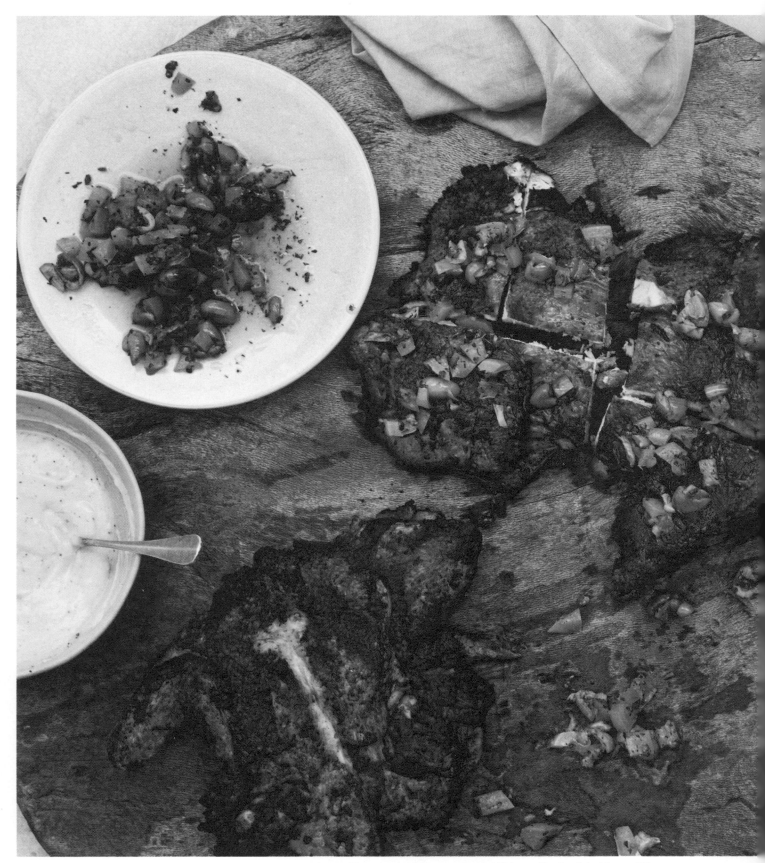

Two-Pan Chicken with Harissa, Preserved Lemons + Green Olives (page 112), served with NY Street Vendor Salad (page 62)

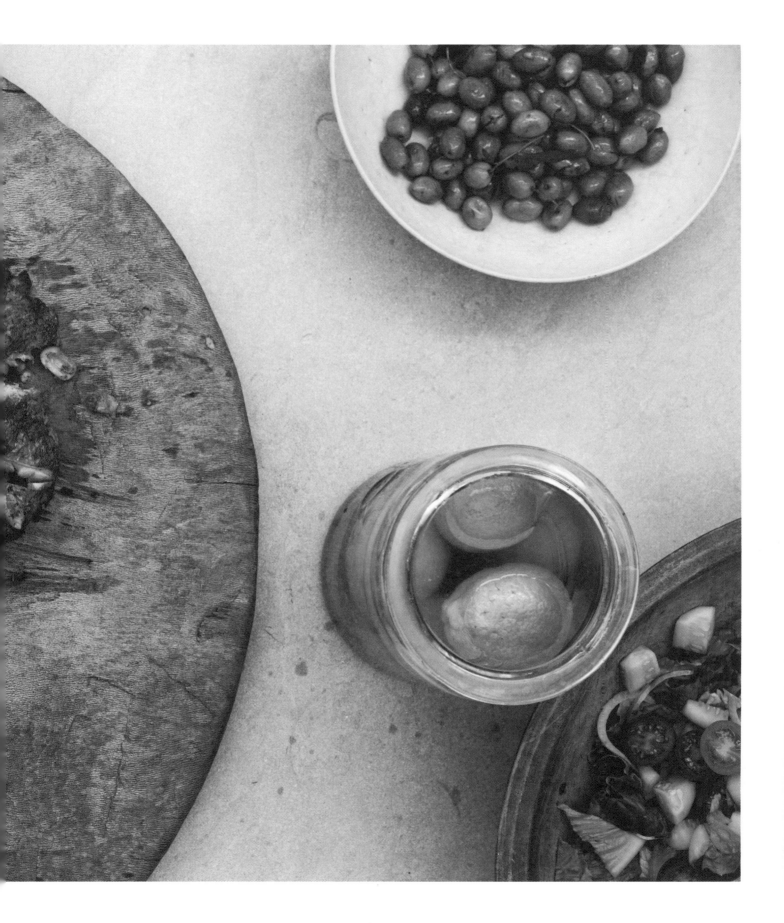

KOREAN CHICKEN TACOS

Julia worked on a cookbook in Korea and brought back some excellent knowledge about Korean spices, rubs, and sauces, which I now use freely in my own kitchen.

While these tacos take a lot of ingredients and you need a bit of time to make each part, the whole dish actually comes together quite quickly. Served with a platter of Grilled Corn, Korean Style (see page 158), this is one of the most flavorful, creative, family-friendly meals around. If you're avoiding carbohydrates, you can skip the tortillas altogether and serve the tacos on lettuce leaves (which, incidentally, is a totally Korean way to eat).

Serves 4

P Protein-Packed

2 tablespoons toasted sesame oil
1 teaspoon gochugaru (coarse Korean red
    chili flakes)
½ teaspoon coarse sea salt
4 boneless, skinless chicken breasts
1 batch Korean Barbecue Sauce (see page 283)
A dozen good-quality corn tortillas
1 batch Korean Slaw (see page 161) for serving
1 batch Korean Salsa (see page 282) for serving
Quick Cucumber Kimchi (see page 158) and/or
    a bit of your favorite kimchi for serving

Whisk the sesame oil, gochugaru, and salt together in a mixing bowl. Coat the chicken in the mixture and set it aside (you can do this up to a day ahead, but be sure to store the chicken in an airtight container in the refrigerator).

Heat a grill or grill pan over high heat. Grill the chicken for about 3 minutes on a side, or until just barely firm to the touch and nicely marked. Brush each chicken breast with a spoonful of Korean Barbecue Sauce, then turn it and brush the other side. Continue to grill on both sides, brushing with more sauce, until the chicken is nicely lacquered, about 2 more minutes. Remove the chicken from the grill and let it sit for at least 5 minutes.

While the chicken is resting, warm your tortillas. Thinly slice the chicken and pile it on a plate alongside the tortillas. Serve with the Korean Slaw, the Korean Salsa, and the kimchi and let everyone assemble their own tacos.

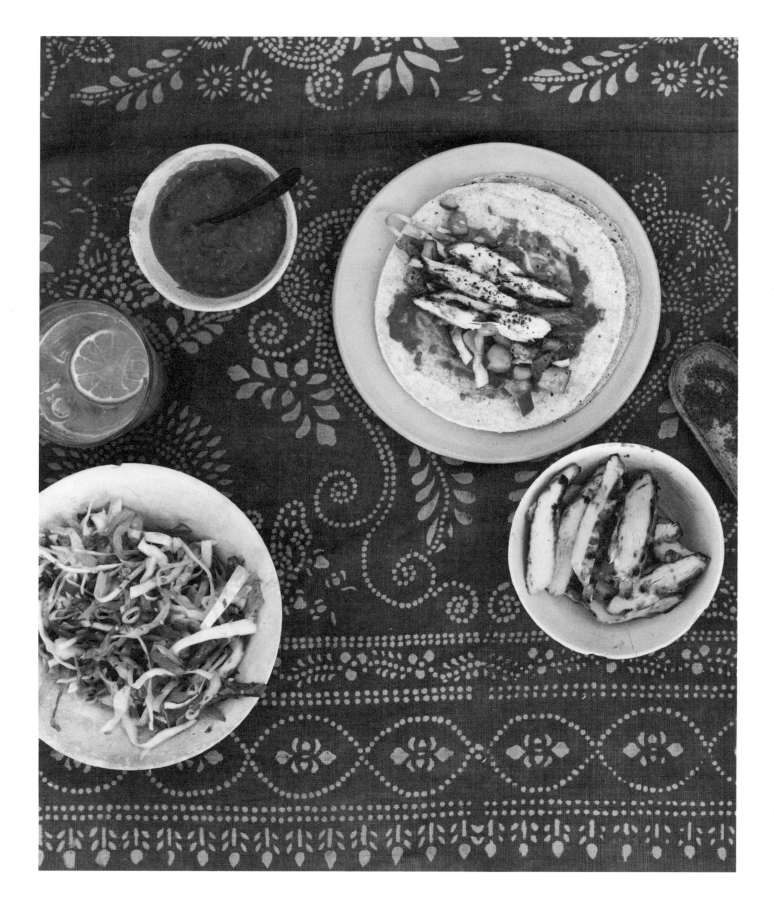

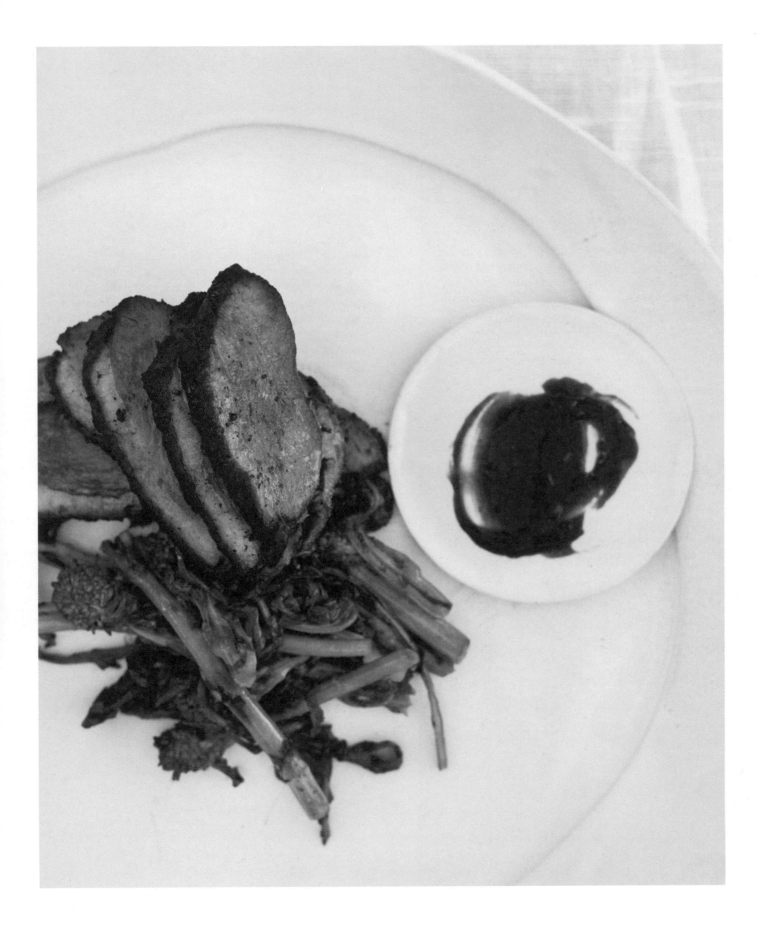

GRILLED DUCK WITH LEE'S HOISIN SAUCE

This could not be easier or more delish. You can substitute other sauces for the hoisin sauce as well. Sometimes I like to sauté a little shallot and then add blackcurrant preserves (or plum, or whatever dark fruit I have) and a splash of red wine or stock and reduce the mixture, then slick a little of that sauce on the duck right at the end. Duck is always so elegant, and because the sauce thoroughly penetrates its dense flesh, you get wonderful flavor for very little effort—a winning main course for a dinner party!

Serves 4

Ⓟ Protein-Packed

Two 1-pound boneless duck breasts, the skin scored
Coarse sea salt
Freshly ground black pepper
½ cup Lee's Hoisin Sauce (see page 275), plus extra for serving

Heat a grill or grill pan over medium-high heat. Season the duck breasts aggressively on both sides with salt and pepper and place them on the grill, skin side down. Cook on the first side until the fat is rendered (don't be frightened if the duck fat catches fire a bit—it's inevitable, but the fat will burn off quickly; just get yourself nice long tongs and have a fire extinguisher nearby *just in case*), about 5 minutes. Turn the duck and continue to cook, turning now and then, until just firm to the touch, about 10 more minutes. During the last 2 minutes of cooking, baste both sides with Lee's Hoisin Sauce. We like duck cooked through, but not extremely well done; it should still be a little rosy in the middle—feel free to cut into it to check on its doneness, as the times vary, depending on how thick the duck is and how hot your grill is. Let the duck rest for at least 5 minutes before serving thinly sliced with extra hoisin on the side.

GRILLED STEAK WITH MELTED ANCHOVIES + ROSEMARY

I don't eat red meat, but sometimes a man needs a steak. I use tenderloin here because it's so lean, but I know the lack of fat can also mean a slight lack of flavor. To make up for that, I use an insanely flavorful, simple-to-make but complex-tasting mixture of anchovies and rosemary to push the flavor over the edge. There are three tricks to making a great steak. The first is to buy a really good steak from a great butcher—it makes a difference. The second is to bring the meat to room temperature before cooking it—this will help it cook evenly; again, it makes a big difference. The last trick is to use your heaviest pan. If you don't have a cast-iron pan, but you do have an enameled cast-iron pot, use that. Or, of course, you can use a grill. Just be sure to get it hot before your meat touches the pan or the grate.

Serves 4

Ⓟ Protein-Packed

Four 6-ounce pieces of beef tenderloin,
    at room temperature
Extra virgin olive oil
Coarse sea salt
Freshly ground black pepper
8 good-quality anchovies
Leaves from a leafy sprig of rosemary—very,
    extremely, super-finely chopped

Rub the steaks all over with just enough oil to coat and season generously with salt and pepper. Let the seasoned steaks sit for at least 5 minutes before cooking.

Make sure your exhaust fan is in good order if you're cooking inside, then heat a cast-iron pan or a grill over high heat.

Place the steaks in the pan or on the grill and cook until nicely charred on the bottom, 2 to 3 minutes, then flip them over. Cook until the second sides are nicely charred, another 2 minutes. This will give you medium-rare steaks. Cook them longer if you prefer your steak more well done. Remove the steaks to a warm plate or a cutting board and let them rest for at least 5 minutes. Meanwhile, heat ¼ cup of olive oil in a small skillet over medium heat. Add the anchovies and cook, stirring with a spoon, until they dissolve into the oil. Add the rosemary and cook for just 1 minute to let it bloom and lose its woodsy edge. Slice the steaks, spoon the anchovy mixture over them, and sprinkle it all with a bit more salt. Dig in immediately.

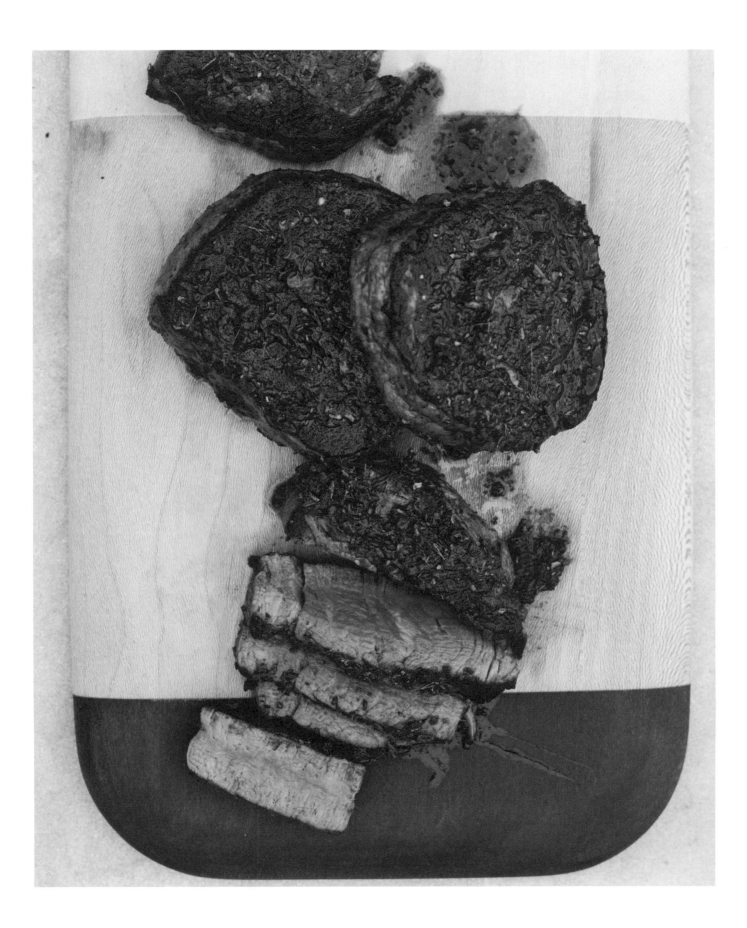

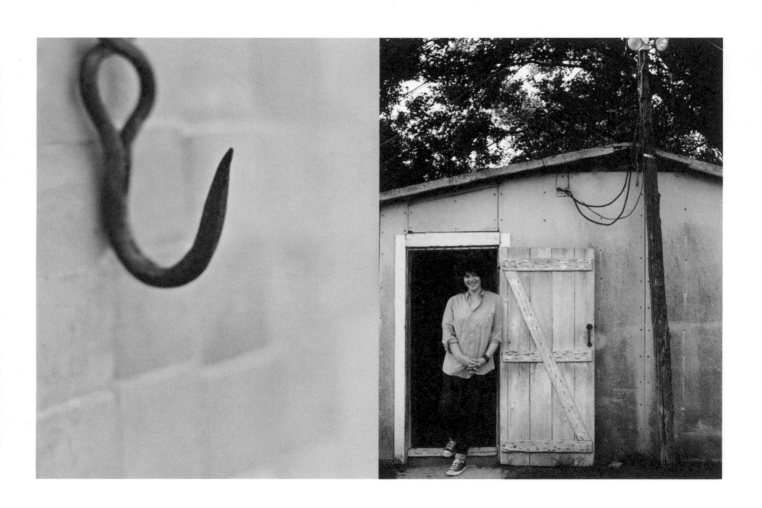

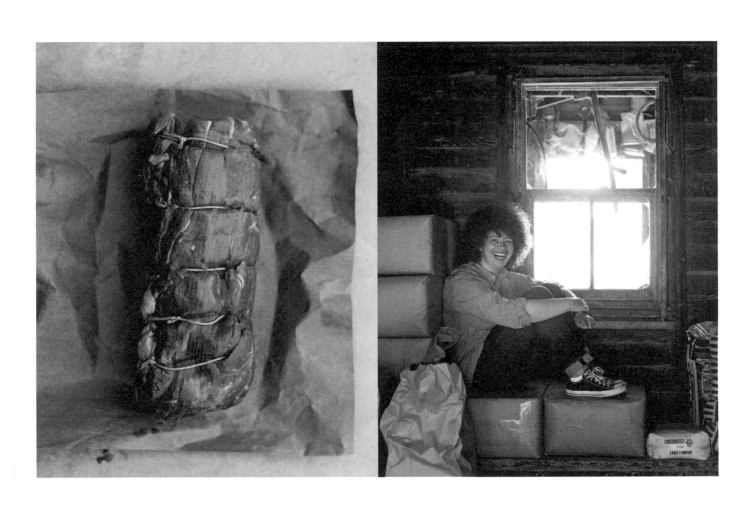

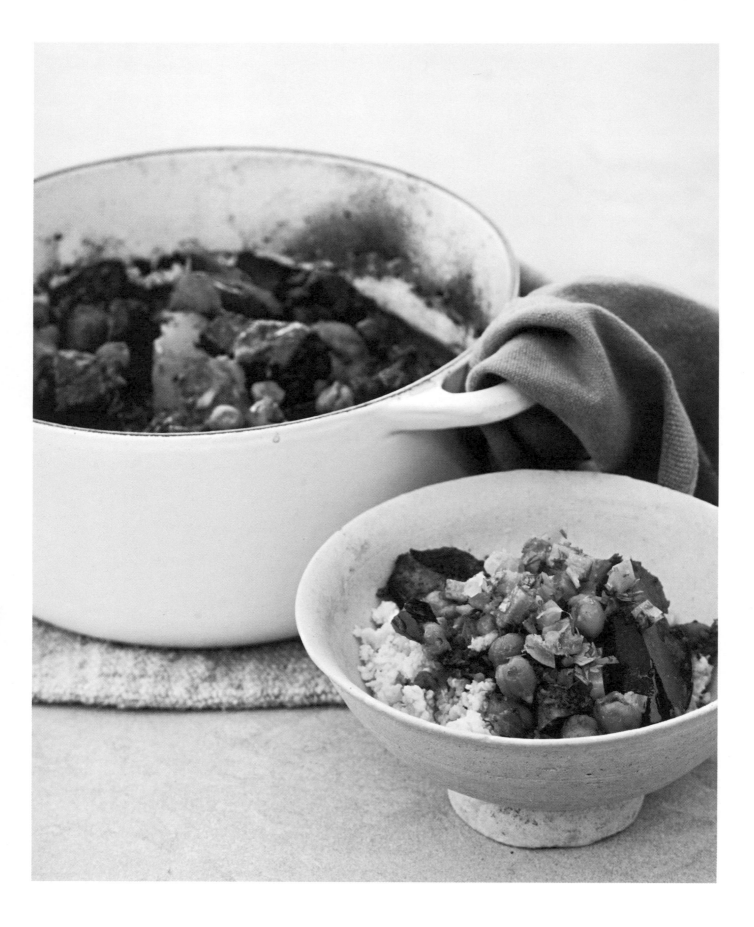

LAMB TAGINE WITH SQUASH + CHICKPEAS

Hearty and warming, this slowly cooked dish makes lean lamb seem the most comforting food in the world. Serve the dish with cooked millet, which has the appearance and texture of couscous with none of the gluten, to absorb all the lovely juices from the tagine.

Serves 4 to 6

E Elimination Diet **P** Protein-Packed

½ cup cilantro leaves, plus 2 tablespoons roughly
   chopped for serving
6 cloves garlic, peeled
A 2-inch knob of fresh ginger, peeled
1 small red onion, peeled and roughly chopped
½ teaspoon ground cumin
½ teaspoon freshly ground black pepper
3 tablespoons extra virgin olive oil
Coarse sea salt
2 pounds boneless lamb top round, cut into
   2-inch cubes
A pinch of saffron
2 cups Chicken Stock (see page 272)
A 14-ounce can chickpeas, drained and rinsed
1½ pounds squash (you can use butternut, acorn,
   or kabocha), stemmed, seeded, and cut into
   2-inch pieces
1 small preserved lemon, finely chopped

Combine the ½ cup cilantro leaves with the garlic, ginger, onion, cumin, pepper, and olive oil in a powerful blender along with a large pinch of salt. Blend everything together until completely pureed. Place the lamb in a large bowl and pour the marinade over it. Using your hands, make sure every bit of meat is completely covered with the marinade. Cover the bowl with plastic wrap and set it in the fridge for at least 6 hours, or as long as overnight.

Take the lamb out of the fridge and let it sit at room temperature for ½ hour.

Preheat the oven to 325°F and place the lamb, along with all of the marinade, into a large, heavy pot (we use a Le Creuset Dutch oven for this) set over medium-high heat. Cook, stirring now and then, until completely browned all over, a solid 15 minutes (do this in batches if the lamb doesn't fit into your pot in 1 layer). Once the lamb is just browned, sprinkle it with the saffron, stir to combine, and add the chicken stock. Bring the mixture to a boil and use a wooden spoon to scrape up any bits that might have stuck to the bottom. Turn the heat off.

Cut a piece of parchment paper to fit inside the pot, crunch it up into a ball, and wet it. Smooth out the damp parchment and lay it over the lamb like a blanket (this will help keep in the moisture). Put the lid on the pot and tuck it into the oven for 1½ hours. Take the lid off the pot and set aside the parchment. Stir the chickpeas and squash into the pot, put the parchment back and the lid on, and return the pot to the oven for a final ½ hour. The lamb should be meltingly tender and the squash should be cooked through but not disintegrated. Season the tagine to taste with salt and serve immediately, scattered with the preserved lemon and the chopped cilantro.

FISH

Fish is one of the leanest and best sources of protein out there, so I cook it a lot. There are exceptions to the rule, however. When you're doing a deep clean of your system, shellfish is a no-no, as are most deepwater fish, which contain a lot of mercury. For this reason, I never eat swordfish or tilefish, and I eat tuna sparingly. In these days of dwindling fish supplies, I look for local and sustainable line-caught fish. It's really worth it. In Amagansett, on Long Island, where my family spends the summers, we frequent Stuart's Seafood Market. It's a perfect shop brimming with the local catch. I stop in for flounder, my favorite white fish, which is perfect for Best Gluten-Free Fish Fingers (page 234 in The Kids' Menu), or local sea bass, which is dreamy baked in salt (see Fish Roasted in Salt, Thai Style, page 134). This chapter is chock-full of recipes, like the Salmon Burgers with Pickled Ginger + Coriander (page 128), that will make you forget you're being healthy.

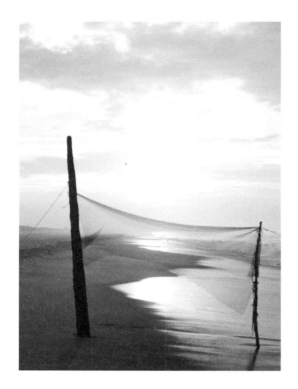
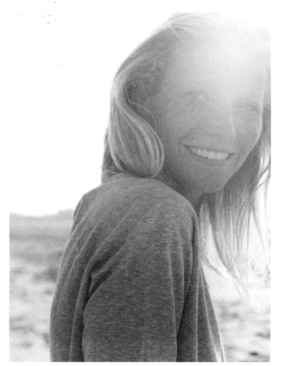
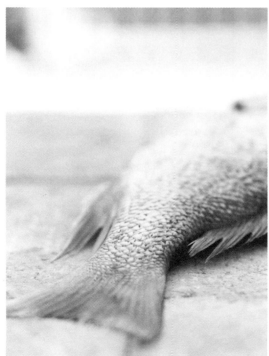
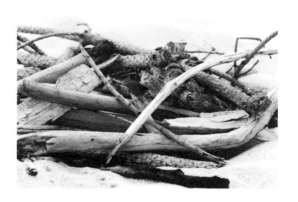

SALMON BURGERS WITH PICKLED GINGER + CORIANDER

Burgers are my favorite food in the world, which is ironic because I don't eat red meat. One day we came up with these and they wrecked my life, they are so good. We serve them with gluten-free buns—you couldn't ask for a more delish, healthy lunch.

Makes 4 burgers

E Elimination Diet (skip the soy sauce and add a pinch of salt instead and skip the Sriracha Mayo)
P Protein-Packed

1 pound salmon fillet, skin discarded, cut into
    1-inch cubes
2 tablespoons drained pickled ginger
½ small red onion, roughly chopped
⅓ cup cilantro leaves (from about 8 leafy sprigs)
2 teaspoons soy sauce
2 teaspoons toasted sesame oil
½ teaspoon coarse sea salt
¼ teaspoon freshly ground black pepper
2 tablespoons vegetable oil
Sriracha Mayo (see page 283) for serving

Place the salmon on a sheet pan or a plate and stick it in the freezer for 15 minutes, just until it gets very cold but isn't frozen solid. While you're at it, place the bowl and blade from your food processor in the freezer, too. Blitz the ice-cold salmon in 2 batches, using your ice-cold food processor blade, until completely minced but not a paste (pulse each batch for a second or 2 about half a dozen times). The cold temperature helps you grind the salmon evenly without its turning into a paste or, worse, starting to cook from an overheated machine.

Place the ground salmon in a large mixing bowl. Put the pickled ginger, red onion, cilantro leaves, soy sauce, sesame oil, salt, and pepper in the food processor's bowl and pulse the mixture until it's very finely chopped. Add these aromatics to the salmon and use a rubber spatula or your hands to thoroughly combine. Form the mixture into 4 patties. At this point, it's ideal to refrigerate the burgers for at least 1 hour or as long as overnight, to really get the flavors into the salmon, but they'll still be A-OK if you don't have that extra time.

When you're ready to cook, heat a grill or grill pan over medium-high heat. Rub the burgers with the vegetable oil and cook until browned and firm to the touch, about 5 minutes per side. Serve with the Sriracha Mayo.

HEALTHY TUNA SALAD

We don't include much tuna in this book, as it's a deepwater fish and tends to be high in mercury. Nonetheless, once in a while tuna makes for a lunch that is as nostalgic as it is delicious.

Serves 2 to 4

℗ Protein-Packed

½ cup silken tofu or ¼ cup Vegenaise
2 teaspoons Dijon mustard
1 tablespoon freshly squeezed lemon juice
8 ounces tuna packed in olive oil, drained
4 cornichons, finely diced
1 tablespoon finely minced white onion
A pinch of ground celery seed
A big pinch of coarse sea salt
A few healthy grinds of black pepper

Puree the tofu, mustard, and lemon juice until smooth in a powerful blender or food processor (if you're using Vegenaise, you can simply whisk together the ingredients). Combine with the rest of the ingredients in a mixing bowl, being sure to break up the tuna. Serve on a bed of greens or between slices of your favorite gluten-free bread.

ITALIAN TUNA + CHICKPEA SALAD

Light, packed with flavor, and super-tasty. I love this salad as a main dish or along with other antipasti such as sautéed greens, grilled zucchini marinated in garlic and olive oil, and grilled gluten-free bread!

Serves 4

℗ Protein-Packed

3 tablespoons extra virgin olive oil
Zest of ½ lemon
1 tablespoon freshly squeezed lemon juice
2 teaspoons red wine vinegar
8 ounces tuna packed in olive oil, drained
A 14-ounce can chickpeas, drained and rinsed
2 tablespoons finely diced red onion
2 tablespoons finely chopped Italian parsley
3 scallions, white and light green parts only, thinly sliced
A handful of arugula (about 1 ounce), finely chopped
Coarse sea salt
Freshly ground black pepper

Whisk the olive oil, lemon zest, lemon juice, and red wine vinegar together in a large mixing bowl. Add the remaining ingredients and season to taste with salt and pepper.

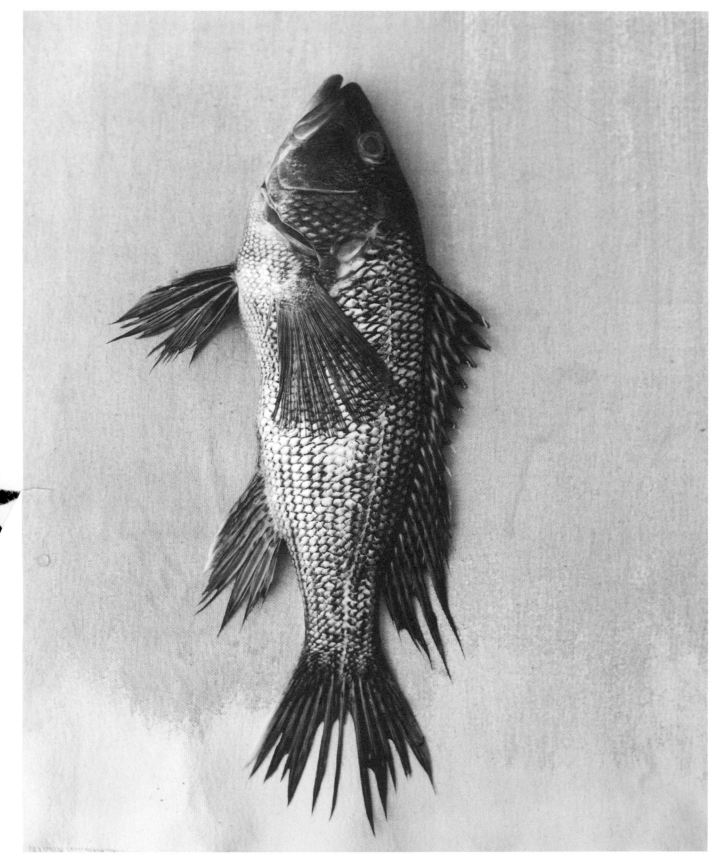

Sea bass

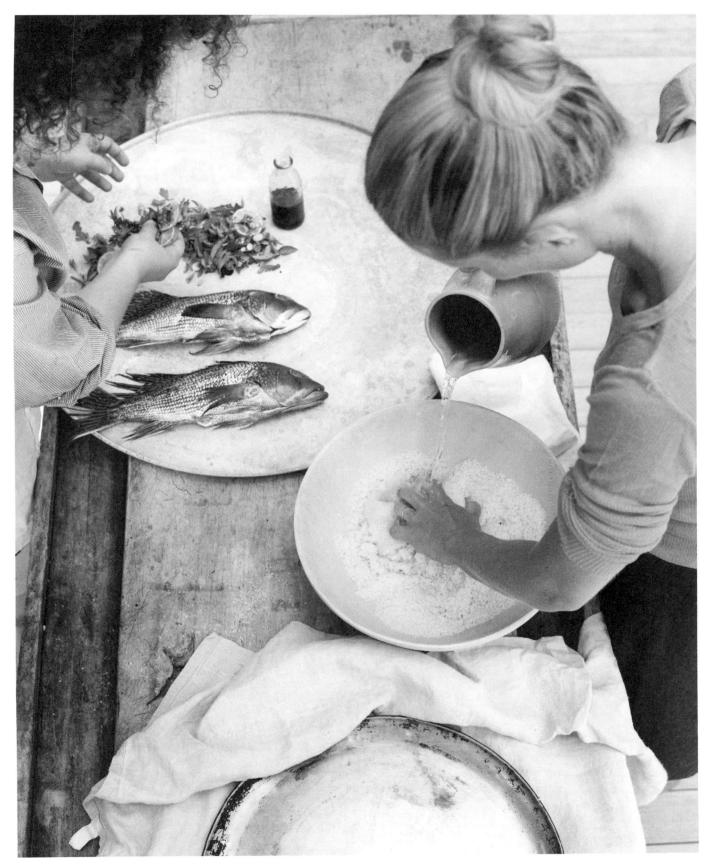

Preparation for Fish Roasted in Salt, Thai Style (page 134)

FISH ROASTED IN SALT, THAI STYLE

This is so flavorful and so easy. Your friends will think you went to Le Cordon Bleu when they see you take this out of the oven. And it's really hard to mess up. Serve it with a couple of veggie sides like Asian Greens with Garlic, Ginger + Fish Sauce (see page 162) and Grilled Eggplant with Ginger, Chili + Cilantro (see page 166).

Serves 4

E Elimination Diet (skip the soy sauce)
P Protein-Packed

TO PREPARE THE FISH
3 pounds coarse sea salt
A 2-pound whole sea bass (or 2 smaller ones), scaled and gutted
A small handful of cilantro
A couple of sprigs of Italian parsley
4 big leaves of basil
1 fresh red chili, very thinly sliced
1 lime, ½ of it thinly sliced
2 scallions, white and light green parts only, thinly sliced lengthwise
1 teaspoon soy sauce

TO SERVE
1 tablespoon soy sauce or wheat-free tamari
2 tablespoons freshly squeezed lime juice
1 tablespoon roughly chopped cilantro leaves
1 teaspoon finely sliced red chili

Preheat the oven to 400°F.

Mix the salt in a large bowl with enough water to give it the consistency of sand castle–worthy sand. Place ⅓ of the salt on the bottom of a roasting pan and spread it out so it's just slightly larger than the fish.

Pack the cilantro, parsley, basil, red chili, sliced lime, and scallions into the cavity of the sea bass. Place the stuffed fish on the bed of salt. Squeeze the juice from the remaining ½ lime over the fish and drizzle with the soy sauce. Pack the remaining salt over and around the fish so it's totally enclosed.

Bake the fish for 35 minutes. The salt should be totally dry and hard. Insert a metal skewer or a paring knife through the salt into the fish. Test the temperature of the metal on the backside of your thumb or on your chin—it should be nice and hot, an indication that the fish is cooked through. Let the fish rest in the salt for 10 minutes before breaking it open with a heavy spoon or knife, or even a mallet if you want to be a little over-the-top. Remove as much of the salt as possible from the top and sides of the fish and peel off the top layer of skin. Remove the top fillet of fish and move to a warm serving platter. Pull the bones off in 1 piece and discard. Put all the lovely cooked aromatics and the bottom fillet of fish on the platter.

Mix together the soy sauce or tamari, lime juice, cilantro, and red chili. Evenly pour the mixture over the fish and serve immediately.

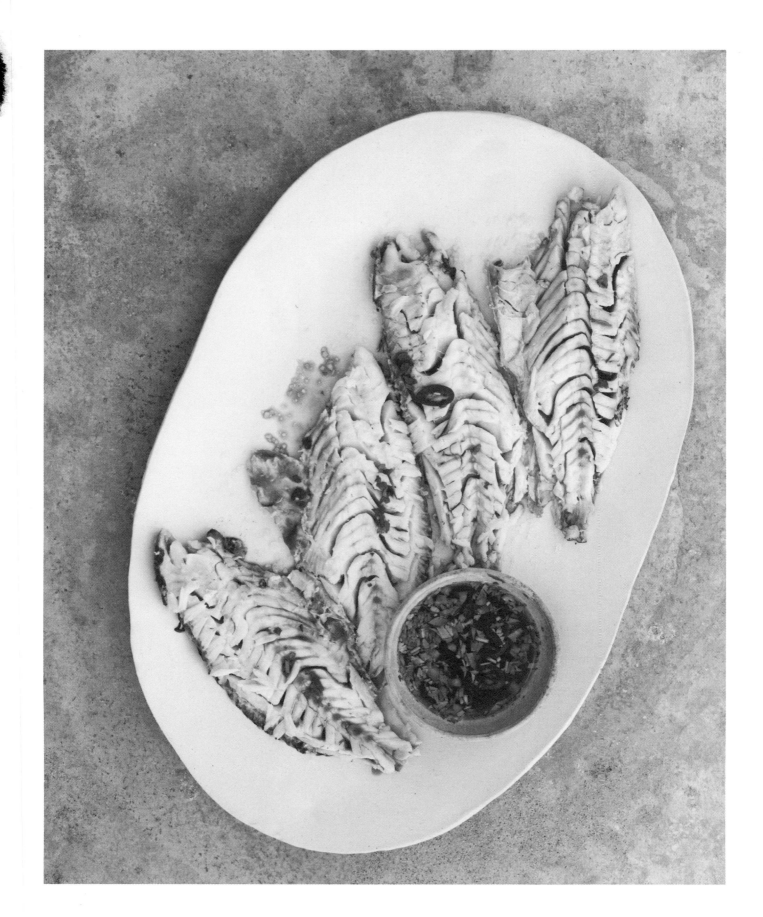

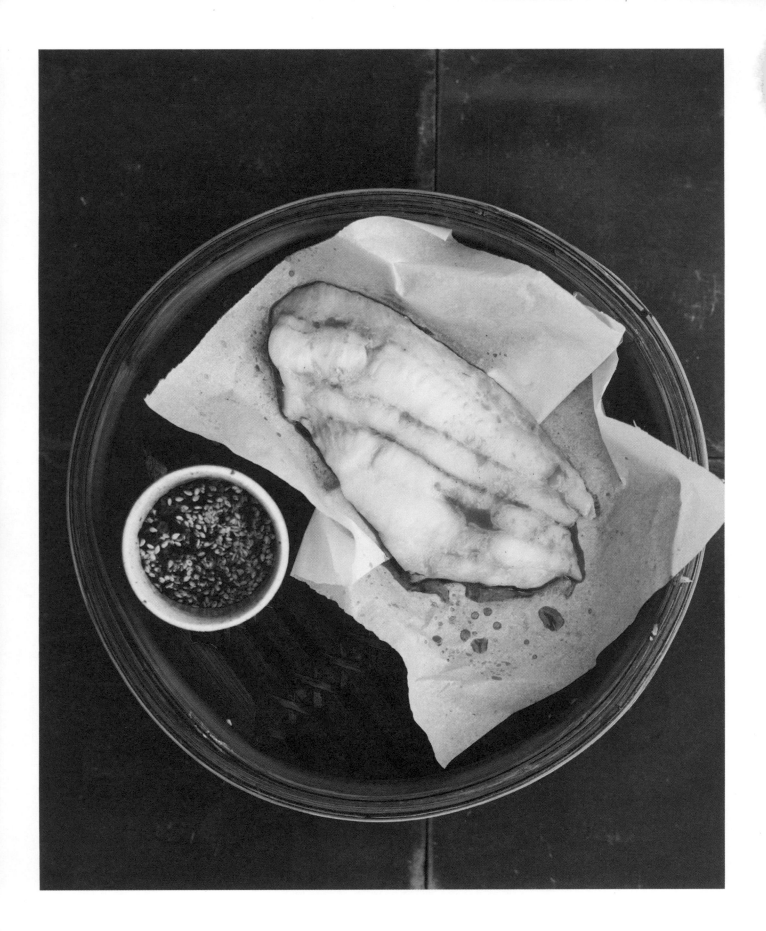

STEAMED FISH WITH SOY + SPICY SESAME OIL

This is the simplest and quite possibly healthiest dish in the world. Serve it next door to some Asian Greens with Garlic, Ginger + Fish Sauce (page 162), maybe a little brown rice, maybe a few slices of avocado—you're good to go. And definitely serve it with a little bowl of Seaweed Sesame Sprinkle (see page 287).

Serves 4

Ⓔ Elimination Diet (skip the soy sauce)
Ⓟ Protein-Packed

Four 6-ounce fillets of white fish (flounder, sole, cod, snapper, whatever is good and preferably swims in water that's not far from where you live)
Soy sauce
Hot toasted sesame oil

Half-fill a wide, shallow saucepan with water and bring it to a boil. Turn the heat to low, set a bamboo steamer inside the saucepan, and line the steamer with a piece of parchment, a few cabbage or lettuce leaves, or a plate (any of these will keep the fish from sticking). Place the fish in the prepared steamer, cover, and cook until the fish is opaque and flakes beautifully when nudged with a paring knife, 5 to 10 minutes, depending on the thickness of the fillets. Transfer the fish to a serving platter and finish it with a few drops each of soy sauce and sesame oil.

SALMON WITH LEE'S SRIRACHA + LIME

This is one of my go-to dishes when I can't think of what else to make for dinner. It's great on top of Lee's Chopped Vietnamese Salad (see page 58) and is an essential adult addition to Rice Cream Sundaes (see page 242). It's also delicious topped not just with cilantro, but also with chopped pickled ginger.

Serves 4

Ⓟ Protein-Packed

Zest of ½ lime
1½ tablespoons freshly squeezed lime juice
1½ teaspoons Lee's Sriracha (see page 274)
1 tablespoon good-quality maple syrup
Coarse sea salt
1¼ pounds salmon fillet, skin discarded
2 tablespoons roughly chopped cilantro

Preheat the oven to 425°F.

Whisk together the lime zest and juice, Lee's Sriracha, and maple syrup along with a pinch of salt. Line a baking dish with parchment paper, place the salmon on top, and pour the mixture over it. Roast until the salmon is done to your liking—I like it when it's just cooked through and begins to flake, about 15 minutes, depending on the thickness. Serve sprinkled with cilantro.

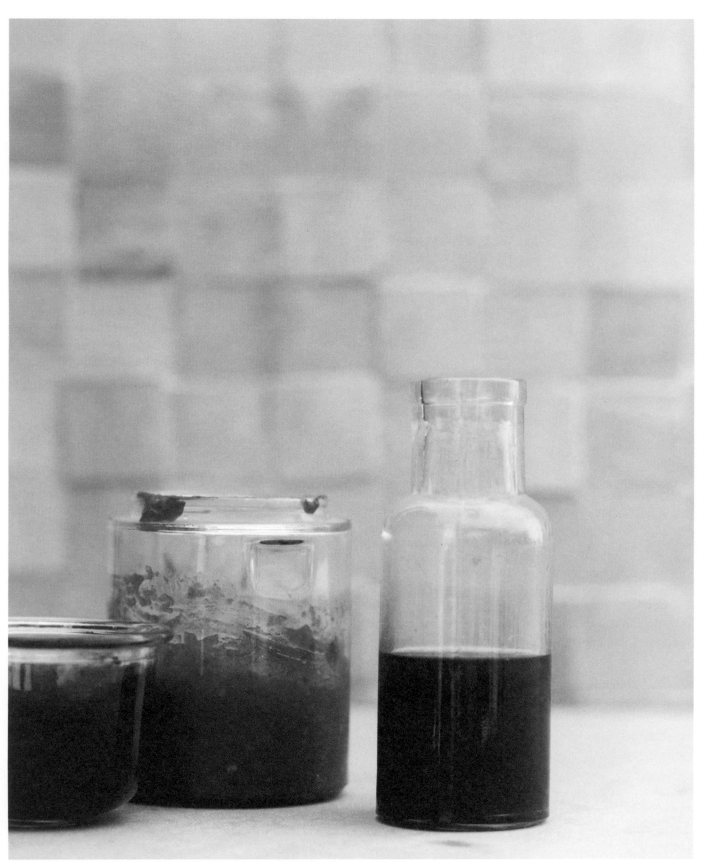

Lee's Hoisin Sauce (page 275), Lee's Sriracha (page 274), and Lee's Ponzu (page 276)

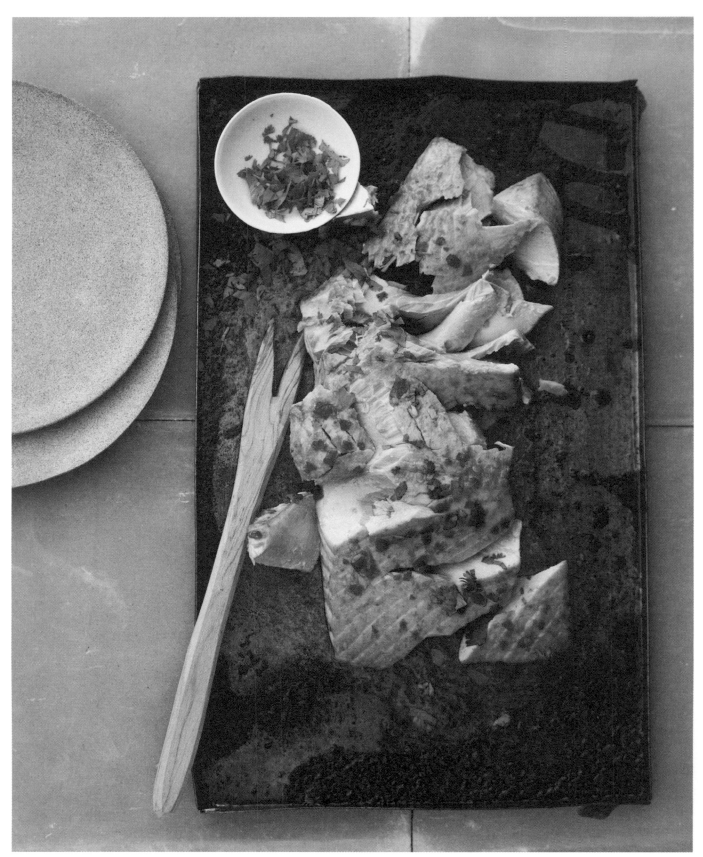

Salmon with Lee's Sriracha + Lime (page 137)

GRILLED STRIPED BASS WITH CUCUMBER + CLEMENTINE SALSA

This unexpected combination came about after a shopping trip at the amazing Santa Monica Farmers Market one day when I had to pull dinner together quickly. It was February, citrus season on the West Coast, and I thought it'd be nice to try using clementines as an ingredient instead of just a snack. Mixed with red chili, cilantro, mint, and lime, it's got a Southeast Asian thing going on and is a totally refreshing twist on plain old grilled fish.

Serves 4

Ⓟ Protein-Packed

FOR THE SALSA
½ English cucumber, cut into a small dice
4 clementines, peeled and cut into a small dice
½ fresh red chili, finely minced
¼ small red onion, very finely sliced
1 tablespoon roughly chopped cilantro
6 mint leaves, finely sliced
Juice of 1 lime
Coarse sea salt

FOR THE FISH
Four 6-ounce fillets of striped bass
2 tablespoons extra virgin olive oil
Coarse sea salt

Combine the cucumbers, clementines, chili, onion, cilantro, mint, and lime juice in a mixing bowl along with a healthy pinch of salt. Stir to combine.

Heat a grill or grill pan over high heat. Coat the fish with the olive oil and sprinkle with salt. Grill until firm to the touch and nicely browned, about 4 minutes on each side, depending on the thickness.

Serve the fish with the salsa and extra lime wedges if you like.

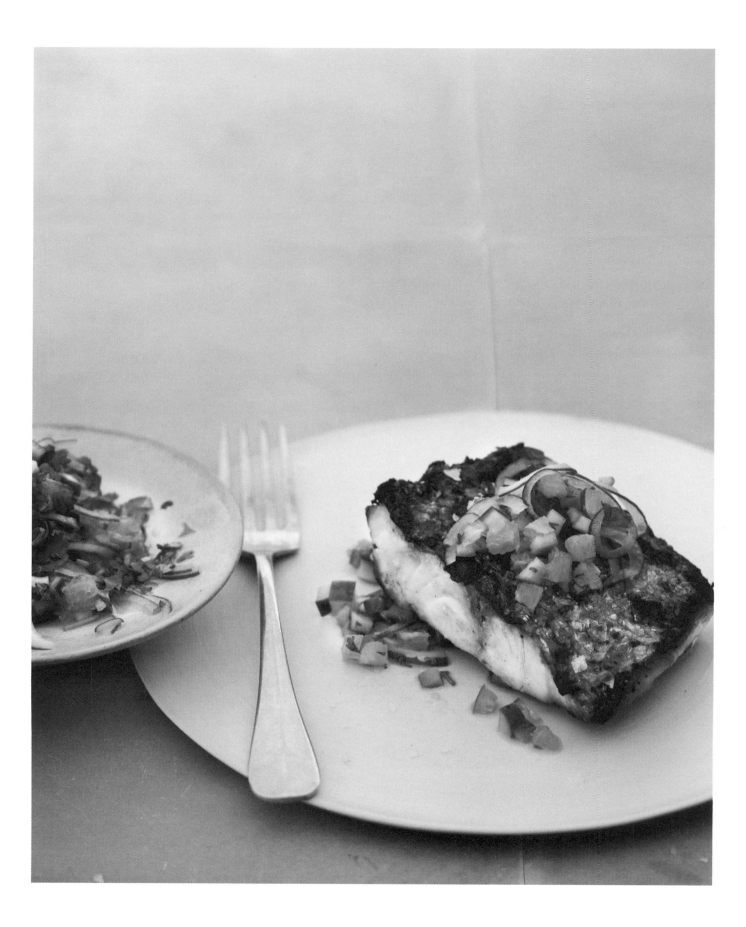

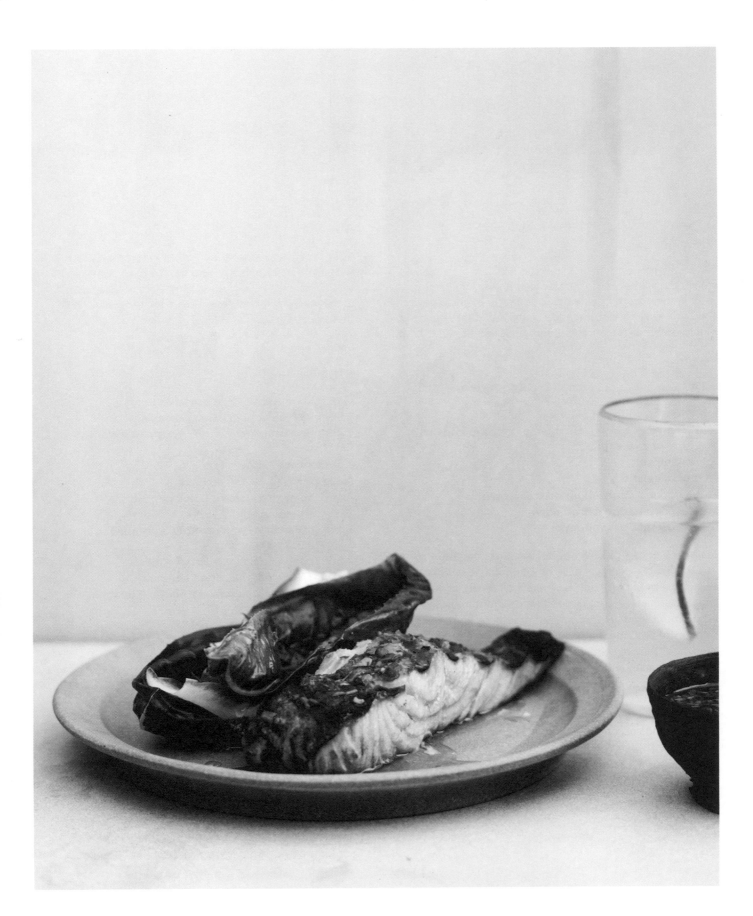

GRILLED SALMON WITH GRILLED LEMON VINAIGRETTE

Fish and lemon are a reliable pairing. Grilling the lemons, which gets all their juice caramelized and makes them taste almost roasted, takes the safe bet to a whole new level. The easy vinaigrette adds accents of depth and brightness while remaining elimination diet–friendly.

Serves 4

Ⓔ Elimination Diet Ⓟ Protein-Packed

Four 6-ounce fillets of salmon
2 tablespoons extra virgin olive oil, plus ½ cup for
    the vinaigrette
Coarse sea salt
2 lemons, halved
2 tablespoons finely chopped Italian parsley
2 tablespoons finely sliced chives
Freshly ground black pepper

Heat a grill or grill pan over high heat. Coat the fish with the 2 tablespoons of olive oil and sprinkle with salt. Grill until firm to the touch and nicely browned, about 4 minutes on each side, depending on the thickness. Be sure to grill the lemons at the same time for the vinaigrette! Grill them alongside the salmon, cut side down, until they're softened and just beginning to char. Transfer the salmon to a serving platter and let it rest while you prepare the vinaigrette. Squeeze the grilled lemons into a bowl (they should yield about ⅓ cup smoky, slightly sweet juice). Whisk in the ½ cup olive oil, stir in the herbs, and season to taste with salt and pepper. Pour the vinaigrette over the salmon and serve immediately.

ROASTED STRIPED BASS, "BAKED CLAM" STYLE

I got the idea to roast bass "baked clam style" when I was in North Carolina during the *Ironman 3* shoot, and fresh seafood was abundant. This is gluten free (of course) and super-delish in a checkered-tablecloth-Italian-restaurant way.

Serves 4

Ⓟ Protein-Packed

½ cup plain gluten-free bread crumbs
1 heaping tablespoon drained capers
1 heaping tablespoon finely chopped Italian
    parsley
2 garlic cloves, finely minced
A big pinch of coarse sea salt
A few healthy grinds of black pepper
Zest of ⅓ lemon
1 generous tablespoon freshly squeezed
    lemon juice
2 tablespoons extra virgin olive oil
Four 6-ounce fillets striped bass
4 to 8 high-quality anchovy fillets, if desired

Preheat the oven to 450°F and set it to convection, if available. Line a baking sheet with parchment paper and set it aside.

In a small bowl, stir together the bread crumbs, capers, parsley, garlic, salt, pepper, lemon zest and juice, and olive oil. The mixture should be the texture of wet sand. Add a bit more olive oil if needed (different brands of gluten-free bread crumbs will absorb differently).

Place the fish on the prepared baking sheet and top each fillet with ¼ of the bread crumb mixture. Drape an anchovy or 2 over each fillet if you're into anchovies (we love them, but we won't judge you if you don't). Roast until the fish is cooked through and the bread crumb topping is nicely browned, about 20 minutes.

CRAZY GOOD FISH TACOS

Fish tacos are always amazing with battered and deep-fried fish, a no-no for this book on many levels. We set out to make the most gorgeous, bursting-with-flavor, healthy fish tacos possible, and boy, did we succeed (if we do say so ourselves)...

Serves 4

(P) Protein-Packed

1 small poblano pepper
½ yellow onion, peeled and roughly chopped
2 garlic cloves, peeled
Juice of 1 lime
¼ cup fresh cilantro
¼ fresh jalapeño, seeds removed
3 tablespoons extra virgin olive oil
1 pound striped bass, grouper, cod, halibut, or other mild white fish, skin discarded, cut into ½-inch dice
Coarse sea salt
Freshly ground black pepper
Warm corn tortillas, guacamole, Super-Spicy Tomatillo Salsa (see page 281), Roasted Tomato + Chipotle Salsa (see page 282), shredded red cabbage, and Pickled Jalapeños (see page 280) for serving

Roast the poblano pepper over an open gas flame set to medium-high heat, rotating now and then with tongs, until it's charred all over. If you have an electric stove, it's best to broil the pepper, but set your oven rack in the middle of the oven so it takes the pepper a bit of time to char. Be patient; you want to not only blacken the skin, but soften the pepper, too—it should take a good 15 minutes. Place the pepper in a bowl and cover it tightly with plastic wrap or place it in a paper bag (both methods help create steam which will help you get the skin off). Once it's cool enough to handle, slip off and discard the charred skin, the stem, and the seeds. Rinse the pepper under a bit of water to remove the last charred bits, then puree the pepper in a powerful blender along with the onion, garlic, lime juice, cilantro, and jalapeño and set the mixture aside.

Heat the olive oil in a large skillet over high heat. Add the fish to the pan and sprinkle with a big pinch of salt and a few grinds of pepper. Cook, stirring now and then, until a bit browned and completely cooked through and flaky, about 8 minutes. Turn off the heat and add the reserved poblano mixture. Stir to thoroughly combine and serve immediately next to a pile of warm corn tortillas and all the toppings.

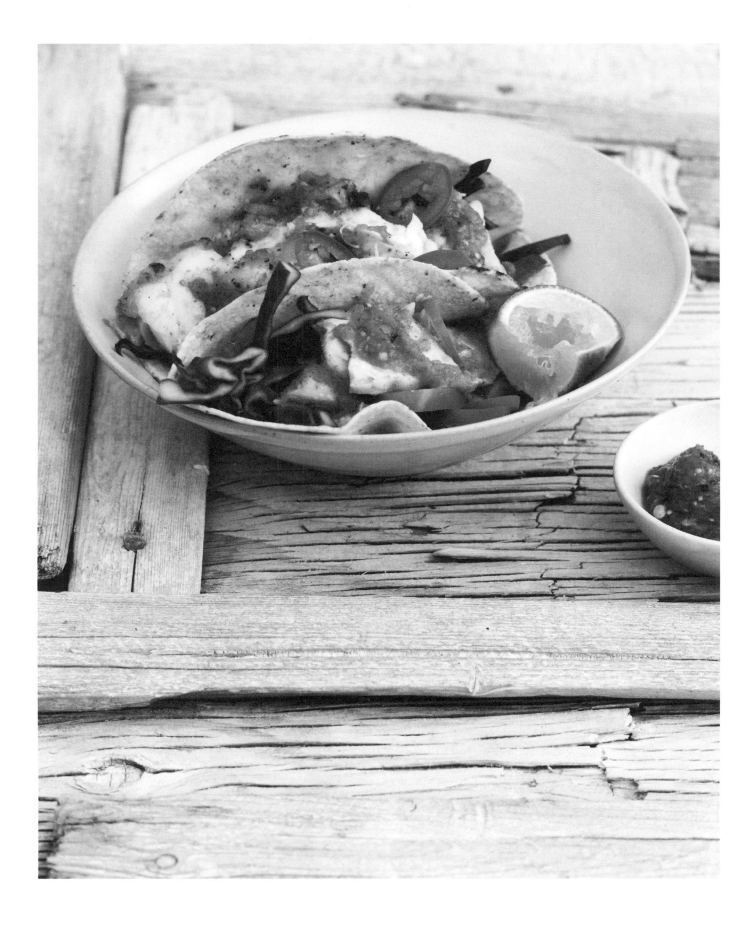

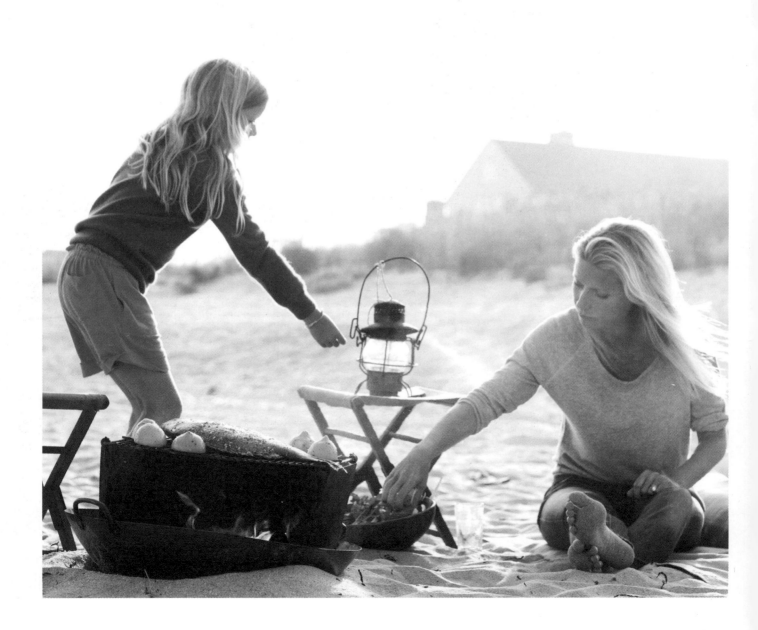

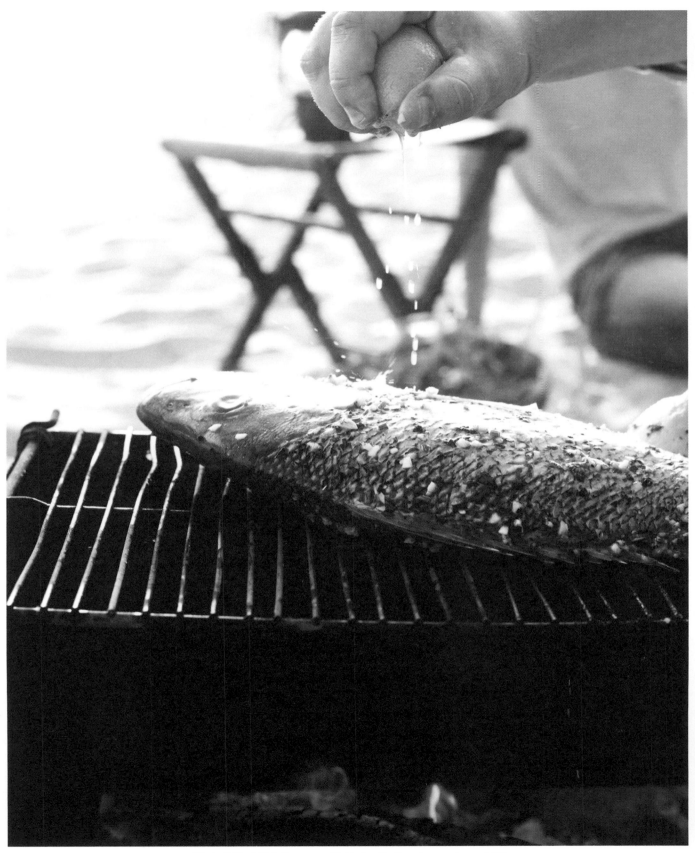

Whole Grilled Pink Snapper with Herbs, Garlic + Lemon (page 148)

WHOLE GRILLED PINK SNAPPER WITH HERBS, GARLIC + LEMON

This recipe is all about technique. You can make it with any whole fish and any mixture of herbs you like—in both cases, whatever is freshest is best. Julia and I last made this when we were together in North Carolina while I was on a film shoot. When we went to the fish shop, they told us they were about to go out to the boat and we should come back in a few hours. We did, and that night we had the freshest fish imaginable, only made better by a few hours of sitting in a fragrant mix of thyme, tarragon, parsley, basil, garlic, and lemon.

Serves 4 generously

E Elimination Diet P Protein-Packed

½ cup finely chopped mixed fresh leafy herbs
3 cloves garlic, thinly sliced
¼ cup extra virgin olive oil
2 lemons, halved
Coarse sea salt
Two 3- to 4-pound pink snappers (or whatever whole fish you like), gutted and scaled

Mix the herbs, garlic, and olive oil in a container or bowl big enough to hold both of the fish. Squeeze in the juice from the lemon halves and throw in the lemons, too. Season the mixture with plenty of coarse salt. Rub the herb mixture all over both of the fish, being sure to get plenty into the cavities. Place the fish in the container or bowl and cover tightly. Refrigerate the fish for at least 1 hour and up to 6 before cooking them.

When you're ready to eat, preheat the oven to 450°F and heat a grill or grill pan over medium-high heat. Set both of the fish carefully on the grill and cook, turning just once, until browned on both sides, 2 to 3 minutes on a side. Be sure to put the lemon halves on the grill, too. Carefully transfer the fish and the lemons to a baking sheet and pop it all into the oven to finish cooking, about 20 minutes, depending on the size of the fish. The fish should flake when you touch it; or you can insert the blade of a paring knife into the fish and then lay the metal on the backside of your thumb or on your chin—if it's nice and hot, your fish is cooked through. Serve immediately, drizzled with any juice that has accumulated in the pan, and encourage your guests to squeeze the smoky juice from the lemons over their fish.

Note: If you like, you can cook the fish entirely on the grill, but we find that the grill-oven combination gets you the grill flavor without all the fuss of turning a cooked fish, and it also helps the fish cook more evenly. Or, of course, if you don't have a grill or grill pan, you can cook the fish entirely in the oven.

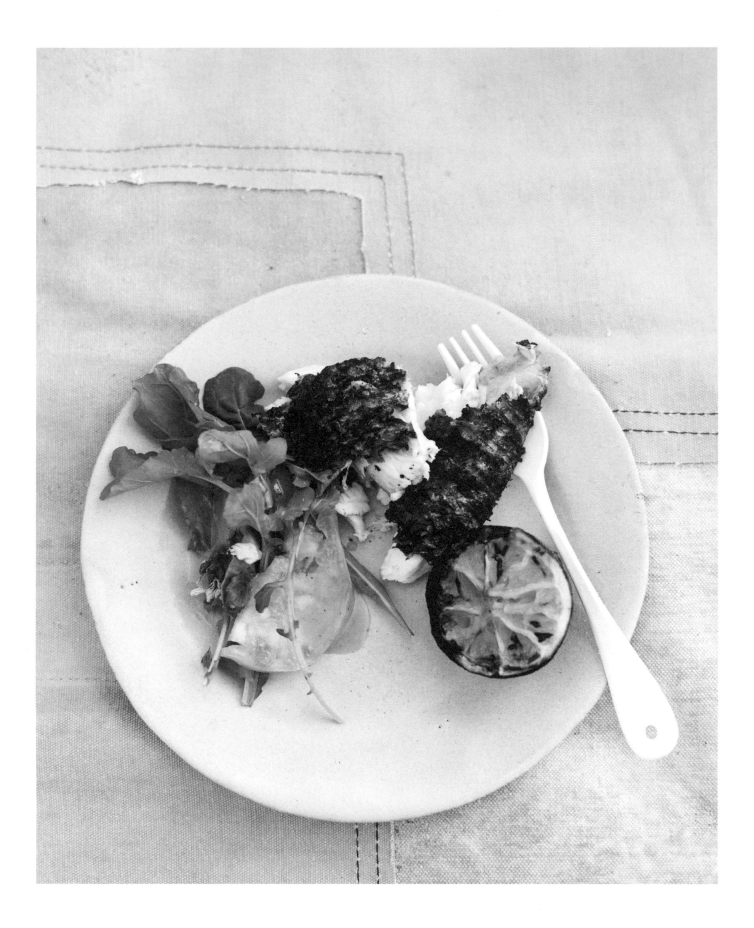

VEGETABLES

Every nutritional recommendation, whether from the most conventional source (the USDA and its food pyramid) or the most alternative (biodynamic vegans), agrees that what should occupy most of the space on your plate is vegetables. Myriad vegetables grow all year long; there's always something delicious in season, and there are a multitude of methods for preparing it all. In this chapter, we've focused on the incredibly delicious ways to bring health and vibrancy to your plate through veggies.

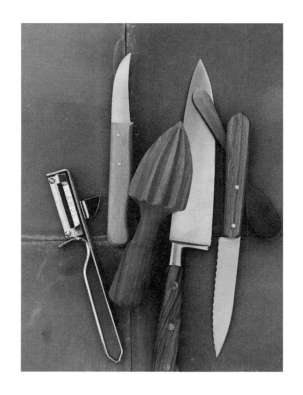
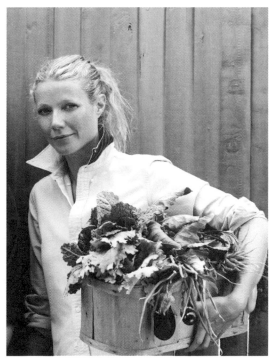
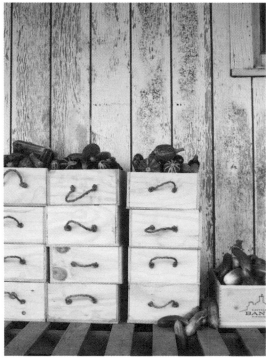
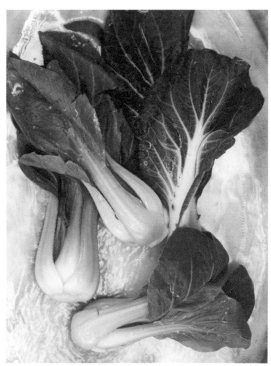

A PLAIN ROASTED SWEET POTATO

Serves 1

E Elimination Diet **V** Vegan

Full of beta-carotene and vitamins C, A, and B$_6$, sweet potatoes pack tremendous nutritional value and, despite their deliciously sweet flavor, are also said to help stabilize blood sugar. A superfood for sure, they're beloved by many of my very fit friends, who snack on them all the time. A roasted sweet potato is a beautiful thing on its own with just a pinch of salt, but you can shake up your routine by mashing your roasted sweet potato with a bit of Chinese five-spice powder, or drizzling it with a spoonful of goat's milk yogurt and topping it with a few Pickled Jalapeños (see page 280). Sweet potatoes are also great with Miso-Almond Sauce (see page 162) and are an essential ingredient in Bernardo's Pumpkin Pie Shake (see page 209).

For the perfect roasted sweet potato, give it a good scrub, prick it a few times with a fork, and park it in a 425°F oven for 1 hour, turning it halfway through. You should be able to slide the blade of a paring knife into it with no resistance. The time might be a little less if your sweet potato is small or a bit more if it's large. Just don't forget about it (as we've been known to do sometimes!). We like to put the sweet potato directly on the baking rack so the skin gets a bit crisp, but we put a sheet of tinfoil on the rack below (or on the bottom of the oven) to catch any sticky syrup that might come out of the potato. Otherwise the oven gets annoying to clean.

GRILLED ASPARAGUS + PORTOBELLOS WITH SHALLOT + SOY DRESSING

This nutrient-packed veggie dish is perfect alongside any protein.

Serves 4 as a side dish; makes ¼ cup dressing

E Elimination Diet (substitute a pinch of salt for the soy sauce)
V Vegan

1 shallot, peeled and finely minced
1 teaspoon brown rice vinegar
5 drops ume plum vinegar
1 teaspoon xylitol
1 teaspoon soy sauce
2 teaspoons water
1 tablespoon toasted sesame oil
1 teaspoon freshly squeezed lime juice
A tiny pinch of coarse sea salt
Extra virgin olive oil
3 portobello mushrooms
1 bunch of asparagus, ends trimmed
2 teaspoons toasted black sesame seeds

Whisk together the shallot, vinegars, xylitol, soy sauce, water, sesame oil, lime juice, and salt. Taste for seasoning, adding a pinch more salt or a bit more lime if necessary. Set the vinaigrette aside.

Meanwhile, heat a grill or grill pan over medium-low heat and brush with the olive oil. Grill the portobellos, cap side down, until quite soft, about 20 minutes. While they're grilling, steam the asparagus for 3 minutes. Once the mushrooms are really soft, turn the heat to high, throw the asparagus on the grill or grill pan alongside the mushrooms, and grill until all the vegetables are nicely marked on all sides, just about 1 minute per side.

Thinly slice the mushrooms and asparagus and arrange them on a platter. Evenly drizzle with the dressing, sprinkle with the toasted sesame seeds, and serve.

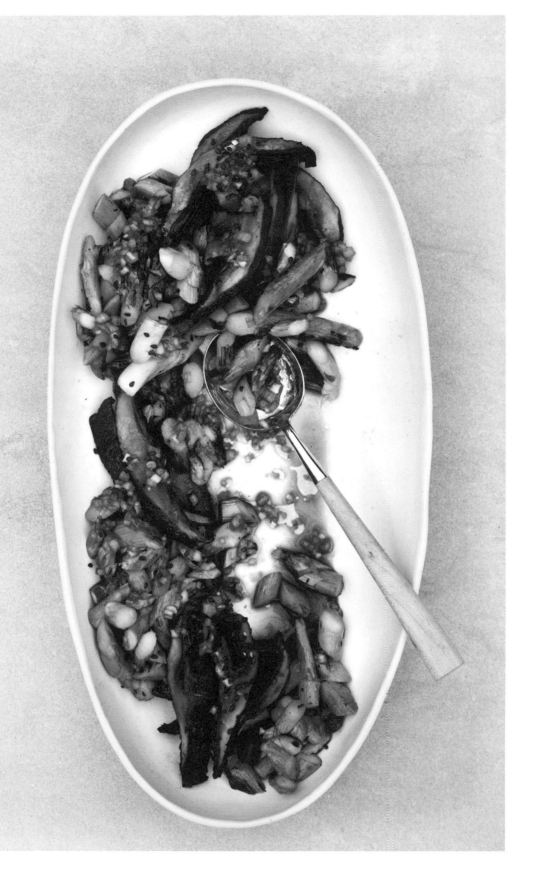

SPICY BRUSSELS SPROUTS

Anyone who knows me knows that I love a Brussels sprout, especially a crispy one. One night at one of David Chang's spots, crispy sprouts came out with bacon and sriracha. This is my version, minus the bacon.

Serves 4

🅔 Elimination Diet 🅥 Vegan

4 cups Brussels sprouts, trimmed
3 tablespoons extra virgin olive oil
Coarse sea salt
½ lemon
1 or 2 teaspoons Lee's Sriracha (see page 274), or
    your favorite hot sauce
½ teaspoon fish sauce

Steam the sprouts until they're just tender, 7 minutes. Once they're cool enough to handle, slice them about ⅛ inch thick (a little thicker than a shred; you want them to have a bit of bite and heft). Heat the olive oil in a large nonstick skillet over high heat. Add the sliced sprouts and season them with a big pinch of salt. Cook, stirring now and then, until the edges are very nicely browned, nearly charred, 5 to 6 minutes. Remove the sprouts to a large bowl, squeeze the lemon juice over them, add a nice pinch of salt, and drizzle them with the Lee's Sriracha and the fish sauce. Toss to combine and serve immediately.

BROCCOLI RABE WITH GARLIC + RED CHILI

We all know how good dark leafy greens are for us, and for taste, broccoli rabe tops my list. The garlic and chili (and the squeeze of lemon at the end!) give it an Italian zing that works great with grilled steak, chicken, or fish.

Serves 4

🅔 Elimination Diet 🅥 Vegan

1 bunch of broccoli rabe, roughly chopped (tough
    stems from the bottom discarded)
3 tablespoons extra virgin olive oil
2 garlic cloves, minced
A pinch of red chili flakes
Coarse sea salt
1 lemon, halved

Bring a large pot of salted water to a boil and add the broccoli rabe. Cook for barely 1 minute, or until it's bright green. Drain in a colander. If you're cooking the broccoli rabe immediately, just keep going. Or you can rinse it with cold water and stash it in the fridge for as long as 2 days. When you're ready to eat it, heat the olive oil in a large skillet over high heat. Add the garlic and the chili and tilt the pan so the aromatics get a little bath in the oil for just barely 1 minute. Add the reserved broccoli rabe and stir to combine it with the fragrant oil. Add a big pinch of salt and ⅓ cup water and cook, stirring now and then, until the broccoli rabe is quite wilted and the water has evaporated, 4 to 5 minutes. Taste for seasoning, adding a bit more salt and a squeeze of lemon if you like. Serve hot or at room temperature.

THREE SIMPLE BEET SALADS

Cooked beets—steamed or roasted—are earthy, often-unexpected bases for interesting salads. Here are three easy ideas. Each serves four as a side dish and can be easily multiplied.

FRANKIES-ESQUE BEET SALAD

Serves 4

E Elimination Diet **V** Vegan

One of my favorite beet salads, especially during the summer, is based on a popular salad served at Frankies restaurants in New York (there's one in Brooklyn and one in the West Village).

2 tablespoons Dijon mustard
3 tablespoons white wine vinegar
⅔ cup extra virgin olive oil
Coarse sea salt
Freshly ground black pepper
1 pound steamed or roasted beets, peeled and
    roughly diced
1 avocado, peeled, pitted, and diced
3 scallions, white and light green parts only,
    thinly sliced

Whisk together the mustard, vinegar, and olive oil in a large bowl and season to taste with salt and pepper. Add the beets to the dressing and gently stir to combine. Transfer the beets to a serving platter and scatter the avocado and the scallions over the top.

THE SIMPLEST BEET SALAD EVER

Serves 4

E Elimination Diet **V** Vegan

In this salad, the simple combination of dark, rich pumpkin seed oil and bright sherry vinegar is both unexpected and dead simple. Love that.

1 pound steamed or roasted beets, peeled
    and roughly diced
2 tablespoons pumpkin seed oil
1 tablespoon sherry vinegar
Coarse sea salt
Freshly ground black pepper

Drizzle the oil and vinegar over the beets and sprinkle with a generous amount of salt and pepper. Done and done.

BEET SALAD WITH SCALLION + MINT PESTO

Serves 4

E Elimination Diet **V** Vegan

Here the bright flavor of mint lifts the beets. You could make this salad a bit more substantial by serving it on top of arugula dressed with olive oil and lemon.

1 pound steamed or roasted beets, peeled and
    roughly diced
½ cup Scallion + Mint Pesto (see page 285)

Drizzle the beets with the pesto.

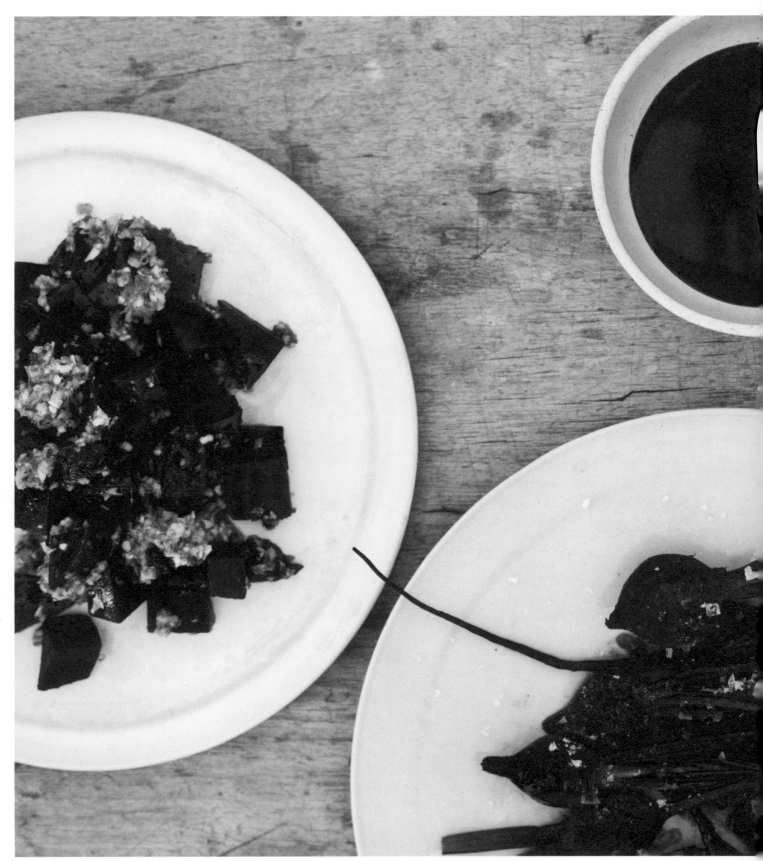

Three Simple Beet Salads (page 155) *from left to right*, Beet Salad with Scallion + Mint Pesto;
The Simplest Beet Salad Ever; Frankies-esque Beet Salad

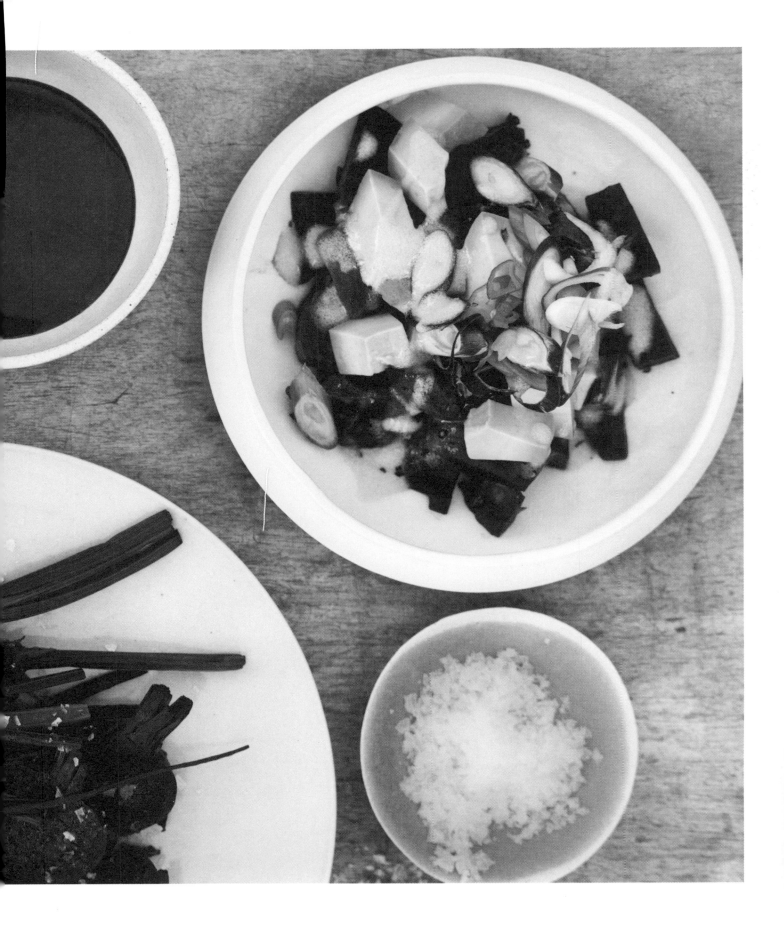

QUICK CUCUMBER KIMCHI

One of the world's best condiments, kimchi is a traditional Korean food that involves fermenting spicy cabbage for days on end. This is a quick and light version that you can make at home.

Makes 4 cups

Ⓥ Vegan

4 cups coarsely chopped cucumbers, most of the
    seeds removed
1 tablespoon sea salt
2 tablespoons white miso paste
1½ cloves minced garlic
2 tablespoons gochugaru (coarse Korean red
    chili flakes)
1 tablespoon toasted sesame seeds
1 tablespoon raw honey

Thoroughly combine the cucumbers with the salt and let them sit for 10 minutes. Meanwhile, mix the rest of the ingredients to form a paste. Rinse and drain the cucumbers and thoroughly combine them with the paste. Pack them into a jar, screw the top on, and let them sit in the fridge for at least 6 hours before eating them. They keep in the fridge for as long as 2 weeks, getting more and more flavorful as they sit, but they rarely last that long.

GRILLED CORN, KOREAN STYLE

Julia traveled extensively through Korea when she worked on a book about the nation's food. She brought back many tips and incredible flavors. This corn preparation is amazing in the summer when corn is abundant and you want a fun variation. It's so insanely good.

Serves 4

Ⓥ Vegan

4 fresh ears of corn, shucked
2 tablespoons vegetable oil
¼ cup Vegenaise
1 tablespoon gochujang (Korean red pepper
    paste) or Lee's Sriracha (see page 274)
2 tablespoons freshly squeezed lime juice
2 tablespoons finely chopped cilantro
A healthy pinch of gochugaru (coarse Korean
    red chili flakes) or your favorite, preferably
    fruity, chili powder

Heat a grill or grill pan over medium-high heat. Rub the ears of corn with the vegetable oil and grill, turning now and then, until cooked through and slightly charred in places, about 10 minutes altogether.

Meanwhile, whisk together the Vegenaise, gochujang, and lime juice and set aside.

Slather the cooked corn with the Vegenaise mixture and evenly sprinkle with the cilantro and gochugaru or chili powder.

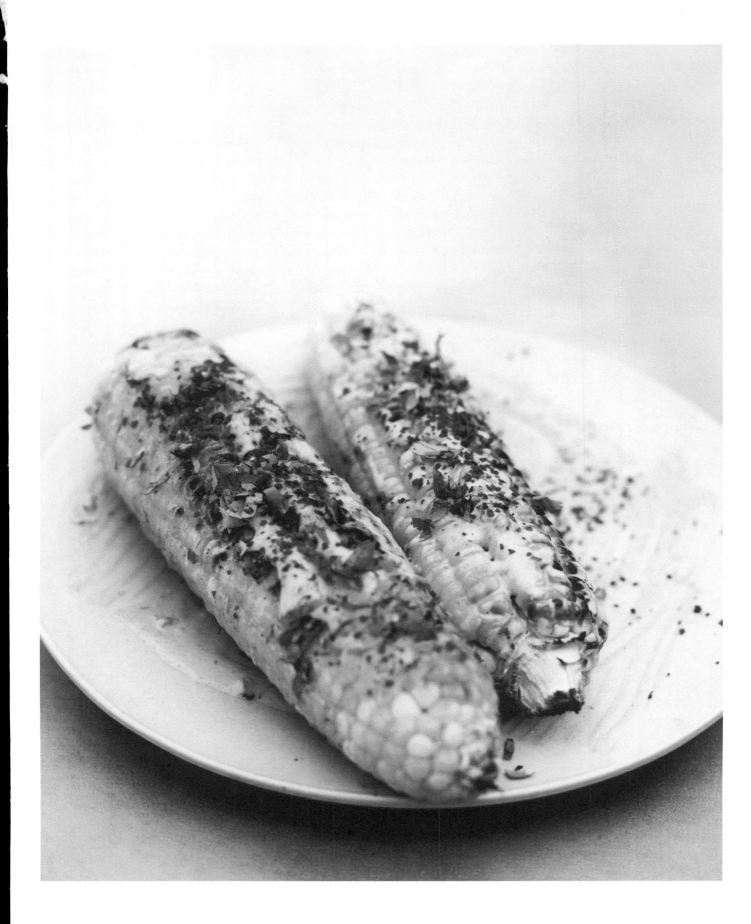

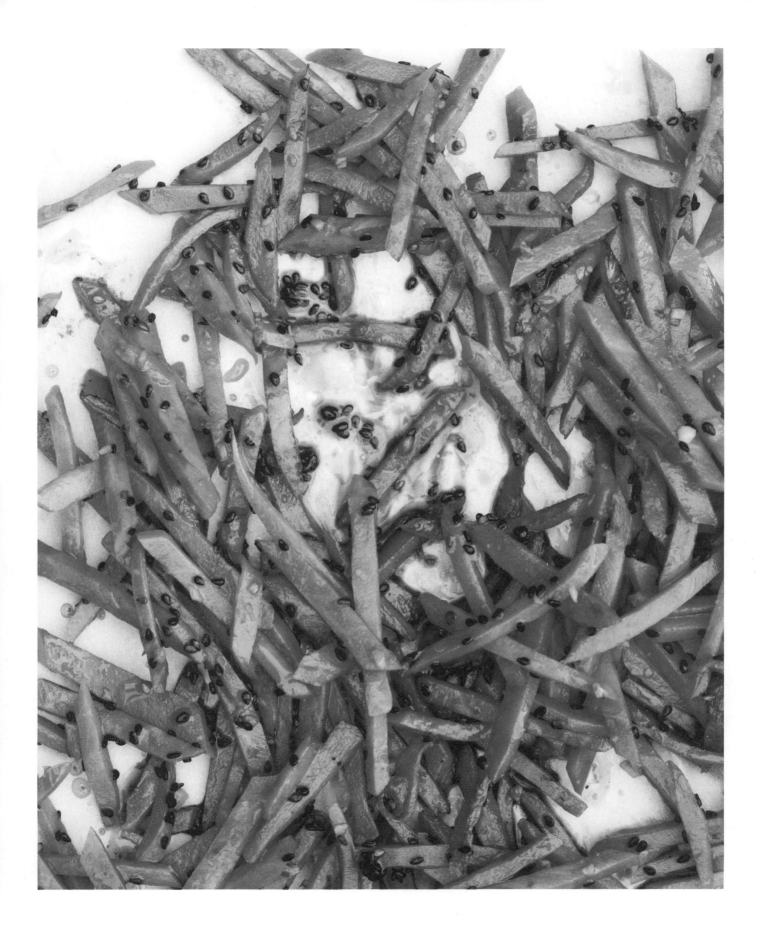

CARROTS WITH BLACK SESAME + GINGER

Good hot, at room temperature, or cold, this dish is a beautiful way to treat fresh, sweet carrots.

Serves 4

E Elimination Diet (substitute a pinch of salt for the soy sauce)
V Vegan

2 tablespoons extra virgin olive oil
2 teaspoons finely minced fresh ginger
4 large carrots cut into matchsticks (about 4 cups)
Coarse sea salt
A couple of drops of hot toasted sesame oil
1 teaspoon soy sauce
1 tablespoon toasted black sesame seeds

Heat the olive oil in a large nonstick skillet set over high heat. Add the ginger and cook, stirring it into the oil, until it becomes fragrant, just 30 seconds or so. Add the carrots and stir to combine them with the gingery oil. Add a big pinch of salt and ¼ cup of water and turn the heat down to medium-high. Cook until the carrots just begin to soften and the water evaporates, 4 to 5 minutes. Stir in the sesame oil, soy sauce, and sesame seeds and serve.

KOREAN SLAW

Originally created for a bit of bright flavor and crunchy texture on top of the Korean Chicken Tacos (see page 116), this slaw can completely hold its own. I love it as a salad underneath a bit of chicken (it's really good with Chicken Burgers, Thai Style; see page 111).

Makes about 2 cups

E Elimination Diet
V Vegan (substitute a pinch of salt for the fish sauce)

2 tablespoons extra virgin olive oil
2 tablespoons freshly squeezed lime juice
½ teaspoon fish sauce
1 cup shredded green cabbage
1 cup shredded romaine
3 tablespoons finely diced red onion
2 scallions, white and light green parts only,
     thinly sliced
3 tablespoons roughly chopped cilantro
2 teaspoons toasted sesame seeds

Whisk together the olive oil, lime juice, and fish sauce in a large mixing bowl. Add the rest of the ingredients and allow the slaw to sit for at least 10 minutes and as long as 6 hours before serving.

ASPARAGUS OR SPINACH OR JUST ABOUT ANYTHING WITH MISO-ALMOND SAUCE

This is so easy, it's a joke. Depending on the brands of almond butter and miso paste, you may want to play around with the proportions. The idea is to have the flavors in equal balance. It makes veggies so special.

Serves 4

E Elimination Diet **V** Vegan

2 tablespoons white miso paste
2 tablespoons raw almond butter (or 2 teaspoons toasted almond butter)
¼ cup boiling water
Coarse sea salt
2 bunches of asparagus or whatever vegetable you're rocking
1 teaspoon toasted black or white sesame seeds
½ teaspoon gochugaru (coarse Korean red chili flakes) or Japanese togarashi (a blend of chilis and other seasonings) or Aleppo pepper, if desired

Whisk together the miso paste, almond butter, and boiling water. Season to taste with salt and set aside.

Steam the asparagus for 3 minutes (or steam some spinach, or dice a sweet potato or some peeled squash and toss with olive oil and roast in a hot oven until soft—the list goes on and on and on). Arrange the asparagus (or whatever) on a platter. Drizzle the sauce over the vegetables, sprinkle with sesame seeds and gochugaru or other chili powder, if desired, and serve.

ASIAN GREENS WITH GARLIC, GINGER + FISH SAUCE

Fish sauce can be scary, it has *so* much flavor. And that's why I love it. Used sparingly (especially since it has so much sodium), it gives an incredible depth to these beautiful Asian greens.

Serves 4

½ cup water
1½ teaspoons soy sauce
1 teaspoon fish sauce
2 tablespoons neutral oil (like canola, grapeseed, or safflower oil)
3 garlic cloves, finely minced
3 teaspoons finely minced fresh ginger
1 pound Asian greens (tatsoi, bok choy, etc.), roughly chopped or left whole, whichever you prefer
A pinch of coarse sea salt

Whisk together the water, soy sauce, and fish sauce in a small bowl and set aside.

Heat the oil in a large nonstick pan over high heat. Add the garlic and ginger and cook just until they begin to sizzle, tilting the pan so the aromatics and the oil get a little bath, all in all just about 30 seconds. Immediately add the greens along with the pinch of salt to the pan and stir to coat the greens with the garlic and ginger. Add the reserved soy sauce mixture and cook just until the greens begin to wilt, about 3 minutes. Serve immediately.

WHITE BEAN PUREE WITH TURNIP + ROASTED GARLIC

My beautiful daughter, Apple, is obsessed with mashed potatoes. She asks for them every day. As white potatoes are a nightshade (causing inflammation) and showed up as a no-no on her food sensitivity test, I devised this mash as an alternative. It's really good.

Serves 4 as a side dish

E Elimination Diet
V Vegan (made with vegetable stock)
P Protein-Packed

1 whole head of garlic, unpeeled, top ½ inch cut
    off and discarded
Extra virgin olive oil
½ large yellow onion, peeled and finely diced
    (nearly 1 cup)
1 turnip (about the size of a baseball), peeled
    and quartered
Two 14-ounce cans cannellini beans, rinsed
    and drained
½ cup Vegetable Stock (see page 272) or
    Chicken Stock (see page 272), or water
Coarse sea salt
Freshly ground black pepper

Preheat the oven to 400°F. Tear off a piece of tinfoil and place the head of garlic in the center. Drizzle the top of the garlic with a spoonful of olive oil, wrap the whole thing up, and roast it for 1 hour, or until the garlic cloves are very soft and a bit caramelized. Set the garlic aside until it's cool enough to handle.

Meanwhile, heat 3 tablespoons of olive oil in a medium saucepan set over medium heat. Add the diced onion and cook, stirring now and then, until softened and a bit browned (but not at all burned—watch the heat!), a good 20 minutes.

Meanwhile, steam the turnip until it's completely cooked through, about 10 minutes (you'll know it's cooked through when you pierce it with the blade of a paring knife and you meet zero resistance).

Once the onions are browned, add the beans to the pot along with the stock or water, a large pinch of salt, and a drizzle of olive oil (about 2 tablespoons). Add the steamed turnip to the pot. Gently squeeze the cloves of roasted garlic from their pockets and add them to the pot, being sure not to get any of the garlic "paper" into the mix. Stir everything together and let it bubble for 2 or 3 minutes just to let each ingredient say hello to the others. Using a wand blender, puree the mixture until it's completely smooth. If you don't have a wand blender, you can puree the mixture in a food processor or in a blender (though if you do that, you'll probably need an additional ½ cup of stock or water to get it really smooth). Or if electronics aren't your thing, you can run everything through a food mill or simply crush it all with a potato masher—this won't yield as elegant a result, but it'll still be good.

Season the puree with salt and pepper to taste before serving.

WHITE BEANS, FRENCH STYLE

Beans are a great vegetarian source of protein. This really simple preparation is beautiful alongside Super-Crispy Roast Chicken (see page 100) or Grilled Duck with Lee's Hoisin Sauce (see page 119), or as part of a vegetarian dinner with asparagus and sautéed mushrooms.

Serves 4 as a side dish

E Elimination Diet **V** Vegan **P** Protein-Packed

2 tablespoons extra virgin olive oil
2 garlic cloves, thinly sliced
Leaves from 4 sprigs of thyme (about 2 teaspoons)
1 large shallot, peeled and thinly sliced
A 14-ounce can cannellini beans, drained and
    rinsed
Coarse sea salt
Freshly ground black pepper
2 teaspoons red wine vinegar

Heat the olive oil in a large nonstick skillet over medium heat. Add the garlic and cook, stirring now and then, until it just begins to turn toasty and brown, 3 to 4 minutes. Add the thyme and shallot and cook for 1 minute more to get them just a tiny bit softened. Add the beans to the pan and cook, stirring now and then, for 5 minutes. Add a healthy pinch of salt, a few grinds of pepper, and the vinegar and cook for 5 more minutes, just to let all the ingredients sink into each other. Taste for seasoning; add more salt, pepper, or vinegar if you like.

LEE'S BRAISED DAIKON

Daikon root is a Japanese radish that resembles a giant white carrot. It's milder than regular radishes and is especially good for digestion. This is one of the best veggie dishes ever, brought to us by Lee Gross, who is truly an expert when it comes to unique and amazing ways of preparing vegetables.

Serves 4

V Vegan

2 tablespoons neutral oil (like canola, grapeseed,
    or safflower oil)
1 tablespoon toasted sesame oil
1 daikon (approximately 1 foot long), root peeled
    and cut into ¾-inch-thick rounds and leaves
    washed and thinly sliced (roll the leaves like
    a cigar and slice)
Coarse sea salt
2 tablespoons mirin
1 tablespoon soy sauce

Heat the oils in a large frying pan over medium-high heat. Add the rounds of daikon in a single, snug layer. Sprinkle each piece of daikon with a tiny bit of salt. Cook for 5 minutes, flip each round, and cook for an additional 5 minutes—you want each side to get nicely browned. Drizzle the mirin and soy sauce over the daikon, then add enough water to half cover the daikon (about ⅔ cup, depending on the size of your pan). Turn the heat to high, bring to a boil, then cover and turn the heat to medium-low. Cook until the daikon is tender, 10 to 12 minutes (it may take more time if you have a tough daikon). Turn the heat to high and add the daikon greens. Cover and cook just until the greens wilt, about 1 minute. Turn the daikon and the greens so they're coated with the sauce and serve.

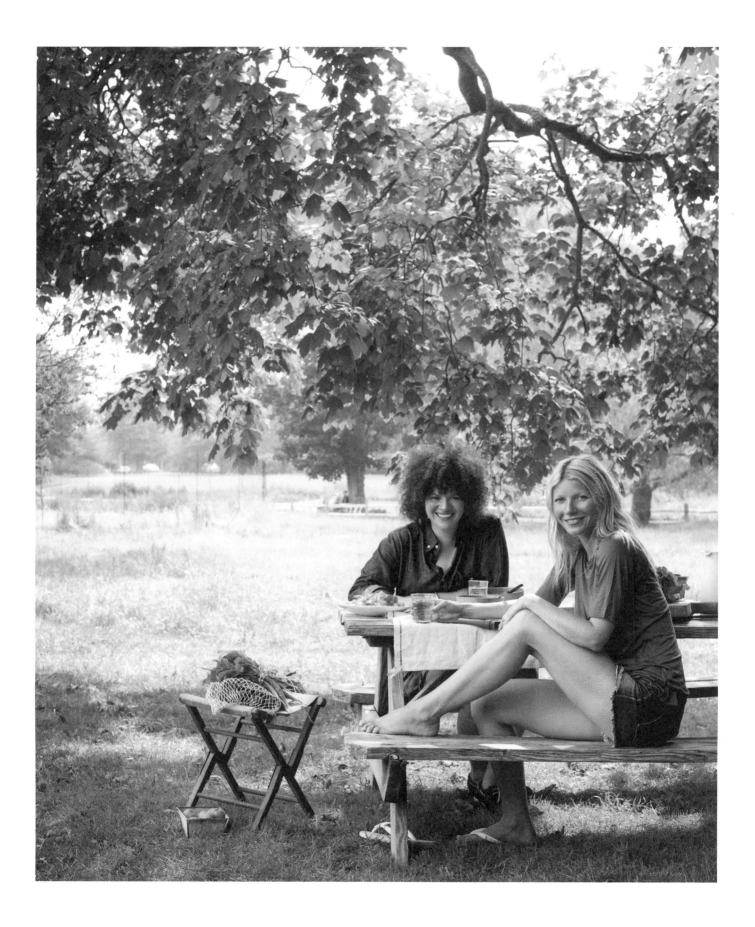

GRILLED EGGPLANT WITH GINGER, CHILI + CILANTRO

Yes, eggplant is a nightshade, so this isn't a recipe for times when you're on an elimination diet. However, when eggplant's in season and slowly grilled, there is absolutely nothing wrong with it.

Serves 4

Ⓥ Vegan

1 large eggplant, unpeeled, ends sliced off and discarded, cut into ⅓-inch slices
¼ cup neutral oil (like canola, grapeseed, or safflower oil)
1 tablespoon finely minced fresh ginger
1 tablespoon finely minced fresh red chili
1 tablespoon soy sauce
2 teaspoons toasted sesame oil
2 tablespoons finely chopped cilantro

Heat a grill or grill pan over high heat.

Using a sharp knife, carefully score the eggplant slices on 1 side in a crosshatch pattern, being careful not to slice through the eggplant. Brush the eggplant on both sides with the neutral oil. Evenly distribute the ginger and red chili on the crosshatched sides of the eggplant slices and rub the aromatics in with your fingers so they stick in the grooves.

Grill the eggplant until softened and browned on both sides, 3 to 4 minutes on a side.

Remove the eggplant to a serving platter. Evenly drizzle the soy sauce and sesame oil over the eggplant and scatter the cilantro over the top.

ROASTED EGGPLANT WITH TAHINI DRESSING, DATE MOLASSES + MINT

Julia here. Someone had given me a jar of date molasses as a gift—it's a very cool ingredient, sweet and rich, with a lot of spine—and I could not figure out what to do with it. I brought it to Gwyneth's house, where eggplant grow like weeds in her garden and beg for something unusual to mix up the regular grilled routine. I put two and two together, and this dish is now a favorite, whether as part of a vegetarian meal or alongside Two-Pan Chicken with Harissa, Preserved Lemons + Green Olives (see page 112).

Serves 4

Ⓥ Vegan

1 large eggplant, unpeeled, ends sliced off and discarded, diced into 1-inch cubes (about 4 cups of eggplant)
¼ cup neutral oil (like canola, grapeseed, or safflower oil)
Coarse sea salt
½ cup Yogurt-Tahini Dressing (see page 62)
1 tablespoon date molasses (or you can substitute regular molasses or very rich, dark honey)
Leaves from two 5-inch sprigs of mint, roughly chopped

Preheat the oven to 425°F and line a baking sheet with parchment paper. Place the eggplant on the prepared pan and drizzle it with the oil. Sprinkle the eggplant with a generous amount of salt and use your hands to toss it all together. Roast the eggplant, stirring now and then, until softened and lightly browned, 15 to 20 minutes.

Transfer the eggplant to a platter. Drizzle it with the Yogurt-Tahini Dressing and then with the date molasses and scatter the chopped mint over the top. Serve warm or at room temperature.

BAKED BEANS WITH MAPLE + MOLASSES

The real secret here is the pimentón. It lends a smoky, nearly meaty backbone to this vegetarian staple, which is great on a baked potato or alongside barbecued chicken. These beans are really forgiving—you can keep them warm over low heat or tuck them into a 250°F oven for as long as 2 hours. They're also even better the next day (when you reheat them, add a splash of water to loosen them).

Serves 4 to 6 generously as a side dish

V Vegan **P** Protein-Packed

2 tablespoons extra virgin olive oil
1 small yellow onion, finely diced (about 1 cup)
2 garlic cloves, finely minced
1 teaspoon sweet pimentón
Coarse sea salt
2 tablespoons tomato paste
Two 14-ounce cans navy beans, drained and
    rinsed
1 tablespoon coarse seeded mustard
2 tablespoons good-quality maple syrup
1 tablespoon molasses
½ cup water

Heat the olive oil in a large saucepan over medium-high heat. Add the onion and garlic and cook, stirring now and then, until they're just beginning to soften and brown, about 10 minutes. Turn the heat to low, add the pimentón and a pinch of salt, and cook for another 5 minutes, or until the pimentón flavor has begun to bury itself in the onions. Add the tomato paste and cook, stirring now and then, for another 5 minutes, just to integrate it with the onion mixture. Add the beans, the mustard, the maple syrup, the molasses, and the water to the pot with another pinch of salt and stir to combine. Turn the heat to high; once the mixture begins to boil, turn it to low and let the beans simmer for 15 minutes. Season to taste with more salt if necessary.

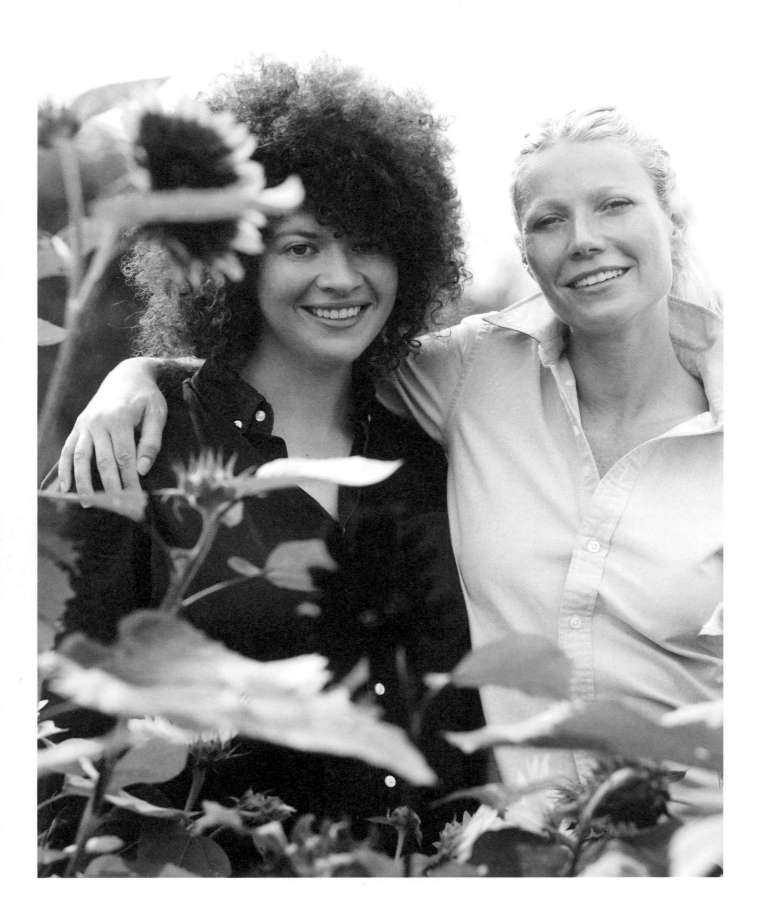

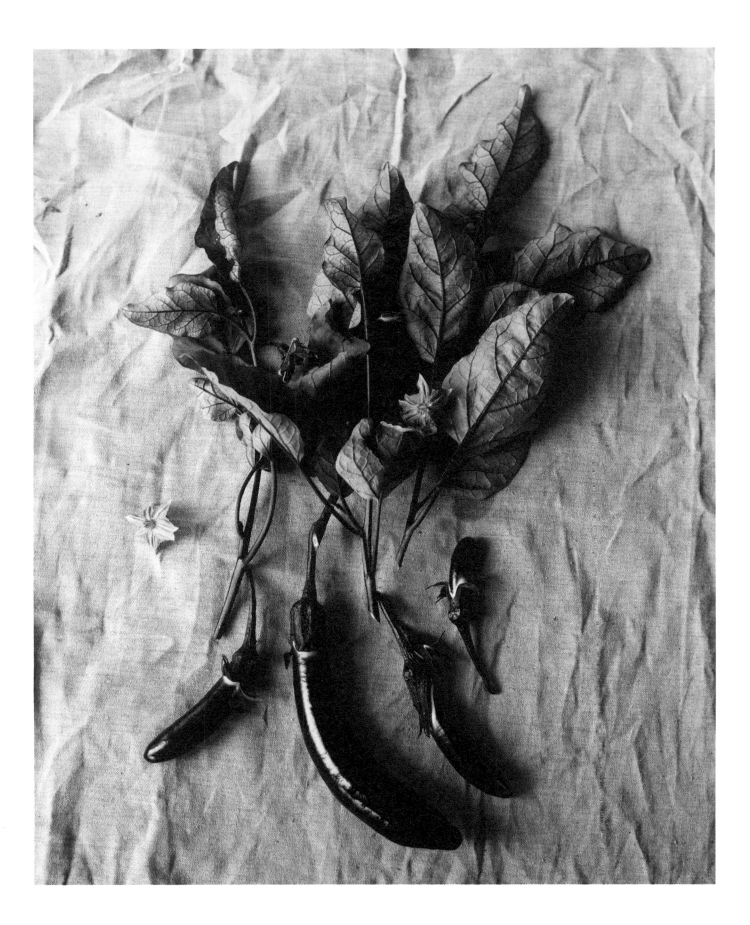

CHARRED CORN WITH SAGE

Corn and sage are unexpectedly good friends. This easy side dish is great during the summer when you're trying to think of a way to shake up the corn-on-the-cob routine.

Serves 4

Ⓥ Vegan

4 fresh ears of corn, shucked
2 tablespoons extra virgin olive oil
1 small yellow onion, peeled and finely diced
    (about 1 cup)
6 fresh sage leaves, finely minced
Coarse sea salt

Remove the kernels from the corncobs and discard the cobs. Set the kernels aside.

Meanwhile, heat the olive oil in a large skillet over medium heat. Add the onions and cook, stirring now and then, until very soft and barely brown, about 15 minutes. Turn the heat to high and let the onions take on a bit of color; it should only take about 1 minute. Add the corn kernels and the sage. Cook, stirring now and then, until the corn is softened and a bit charred around the edges, 4 to 5 minutes. Season to taste with salt and serve immediately or at room temperature.

SAUTÉED CORN WITH CHIMICHURRI

Another favorite, easy corn dish. We created this recipe after we had tested our chimichurri and had so much on hand we were looking for ways to use it up. A pile of corn on the counter solved our problem.

Serves 4

Ⓥ Vegan

4 fresh ears of corn, shucked
2 tablespoons extra virgin olive oil
Coarse sea salt
2 tablespoons Chimichurri (see page 284)

Remove the kernels from the corncobs and discard the cobs. Heat the olive oil in a large nonstick skillet set over high heat and immediately add the corn kernels and a large pinch of salt. Cook, stirring now and then, until the corn is softened and takes on a bit of char around the edges, 4 to 5 minutes. Turn off the heat and stir in the Chimichurri. Season to taste with more salt if needed. Serve immediately or at room temperature.

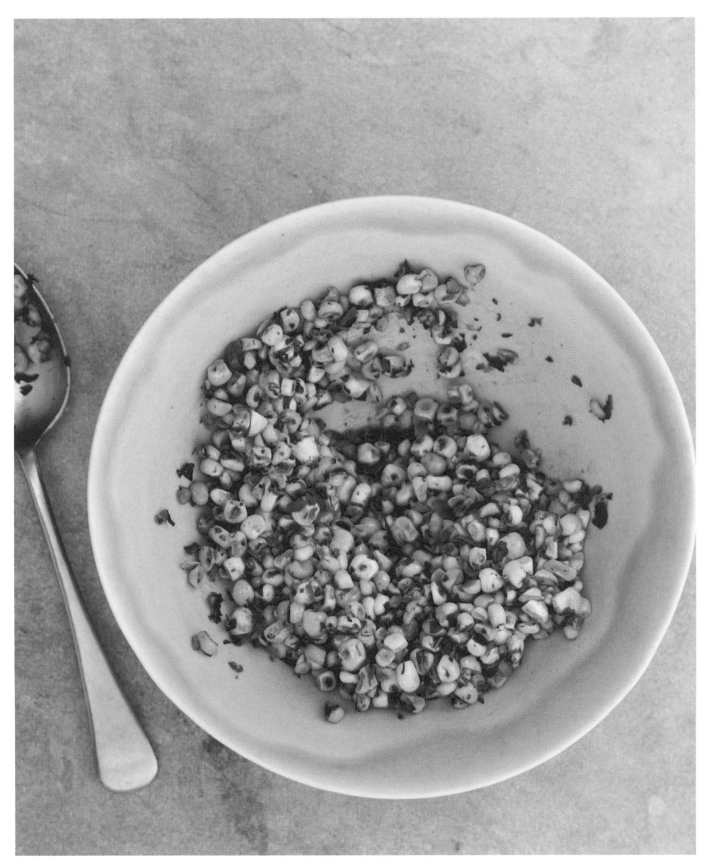

Sautéed Corn with Chimichurri

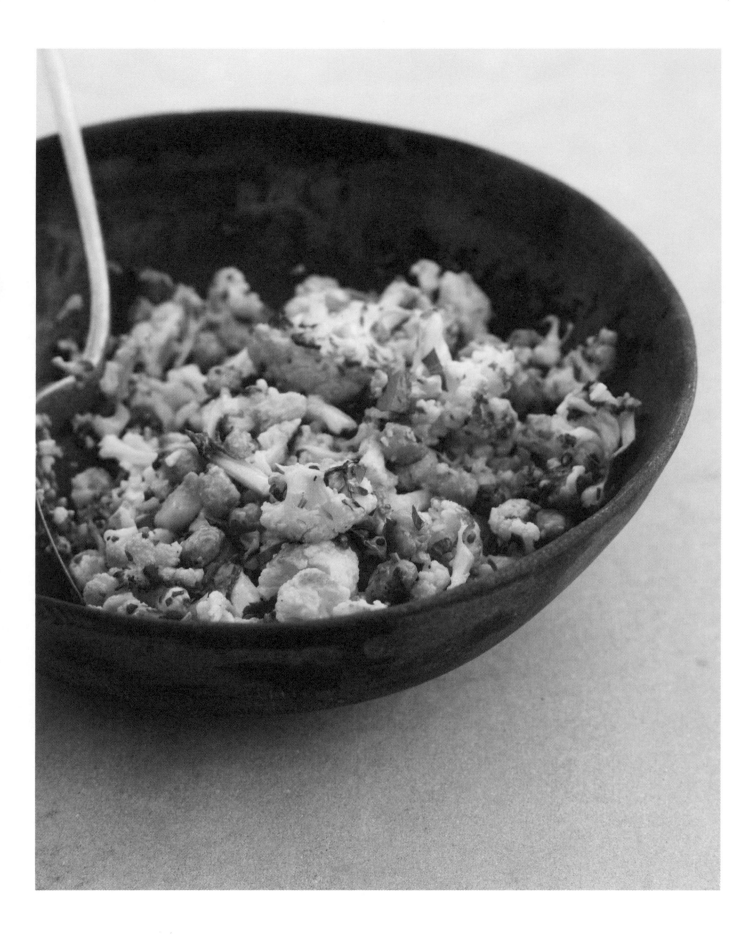

ROASTED CAULIFLOWER + CHICKPEAS WITH MUSTARD + PARSLEY

So good. Roasted cauliflower, with its gently browned florets, is a sweet and deep contrast to the fiber-rich roasted chickpea. This is an ultrahealthy and filling side, one of those healthy dishes that actually leaves you feeling satisfied.

Serves 4

E Elimination Diet **V** Vegan **P** Protein-Packed

A 14-ounce can chickpeas, rinsed and drained and dried in a kitchen towel
1 head of cauliflower, outer leaves removed and discarded (or slice and sauté them with garlic—they're surprisingly delicious!), cut into bite-sized florets
Extra virgin olive oil
Coarse sea salt
1 tablespoon Dijon mustard
1 tablespoon seeded mustard
1 tablespoon white wine vinegar
Freshly ground black pepper
¼ cup chopped Italian parsley

Preheat the oven to 400°F and set the rack in the middle.

Toss the chickpeas and cauliflower together in a large roasting pan with 3 tablespoons of olive oil and a big pinch of salt. Roast, stirring now and then, until everything is dark brown and the cauliflower is quite soft, about 45 minutes.

Meanwhile, whisk together the mustards, vinegar, and ¼ cup of olive oil with a big pinch of salt and a few healthy grinds of black pepper. While the chickpeas and cauliflower are still warm, toss them with the mustard dressing and the parsley. Serve warm or at room temperature.

ROASTED ROMANESCO WITH AIOLI + FRIED CAPERS

Julia here. Once when I was having dinner at Prune, Gabrielle Hamilton's perfect restaurant on East First Street, which I've been devoted to since it opened over a decade ago, I was taken aback by a perfect side dish of roasted cauliflower served with a strong aioli and capers. When I saw romanesco at the market one day—that funny-looking vegetable that looks like a cauliflower on acid—I thought I'd give her amazing combination a try. Vegan friends go nuts for this.

Serves 4

 Vegan

1 head of romanesco or cauliflower, outer leaves
    removed and discarded (or slice and sauté
    them with garlic—they're surprisingly
    delicious!), cut into bite-sized florets
Extra virgin olive oil
Coarse sea salt
¼ cup capers, rinsed and dried on a paper towel
½ cup Vegenaise
1 garlic clove, very finely minced
1 tablespoon freshly squeezed lemon juice
¼ cup chopped Italian parsley

Preheat the oven to 425°F and set the rack in the middle. Line a baking sheet with parchment paper, place the romanesco or cauliflower on it, and drizzle with 3 tablespoons of olive oil. Sprinkle evenly with a nice pinch of salt and roast, stirring now and then, until each floret is softened and a bit charred in places, about ½ hour.

Meanwhile, heat ½ inch of olive oil in a small skillet set over high heat and fry the capers, stirring once or twice, until really crispy, about 2 minutes (be very careful when doing this, as they tend to pop a bit). Remove the capers from the hot oil with a slotted spoon, transfer them to a plate, and set them aside.

Whisk together the Vegenaise, garlic, and lemon juice to make aioli, and season to taste with salt. Transfer the roasted romanesco or cauliflower to a platter, drizzle with the aioli, and scatter the fried capers and the chopped parsley over the top. Serve warm or at room temperature.

ROASTED LEEKS, TWO WAYS

I used to encounter braised leeks in France when I lived there, and I marveled at how sweet they were when they had been caramelized. I hardly ever make a roast chicken without leeks on the side. Here are two preparations using roasted, caramelized leeks that are sure to please.

Serves 4

V Vegan (both versions)

6 leeks, white and light green parts only, thoroughly washed and cut in half lengthwise
3 tablespoons extra virgin olive oil
Coarse sea salt
Romesco Sauce or Shallot Vinaigrette for serving

Preheat the oven to 425°F and line a baking sheet with parchment. Line the leeks up on the baking sheet and drizzle with the olive oil—use your hands to make sure they're completely coated. Sprinkle with a big pinch of salt and roast until they're softened and a bit browned, about 20 minutes. Serve with Romesco Sauce or Shallot Vinaigrette, and eat warm or at room temperature.

ROMESCO SAUCE

Makes ⅓ cup

1 roasted red bell pepper
1 small garlic clove, crushed
3 tablespoons toasted, blanched almonds (cooled)
1 teaspoon sherry vinegar
3 tablespoons extra virgin olive oil
Coarse sea salt
Freshly ground black pepper

Roast the pepper over an open gas flame set to medium-high heat, rotating now and then with tongs, until it's charred all over. If you have an electric stove, it's best to broil the pepper, but set your oven rack in the middle of the oven so it takes the pepper a bit of time to char. Be patient; you want to not only blacken the skin, but soften the pepper, too—it should take a good 15 minutes. Place the pepper in a bowl and cover it tightly with plastic wrap or place it in a paper bag (both methods help create steam which will help you get the skin off). Once it's cool enough to handle, slip off and discard the charred skin, the stem, and the seeds. Rinse the pepper under a bit of water to remove the last charred bits, then puree the pepper along with the garlic, almonds, sherry vinegar, and olive oil. Season to taste with salt and pepper.

SHALLOT VINAIGRETTE

Makes ¼ cup

1 teaspoon Dijon mustard
1 teaspoon xylitol or good-quality maple syrup
1 tablespoon white wine vinegar
3 tablespoons extra virgin olive oil
1 tablespoon very finely diced shallot (1 small shallot)
Coarse sea salt
Freshly ground black pepper

Whisk together the mustard, xylitol, and white wine vinegar. While whisking, slowly pour in the olive oil until it's emulsified. Stir in the shallot. Season to taste with salt and pepper.

GRAINS

Every single nutritionist, doctor, and health-conscious person I have ever come across recommends that organic whole grains (in addition to vegetables!) be the center of your plate. There are so many beautiful varieties. I stay away from the ones containing gluten, as those same folks listed above seem to concur that it is tough on the system and that many of us are at best intolerant of it and at worst allergic to it. Sometimes when my family is not eating pasta, bread, or processed grains like white rice, we're left with that specific hunger that comes with avoiding carbs. So, if Julia and I do say so ourselves, we have created a whole bunch of incredibly satisfying, incredibly good-for-you grain-based recipes that will leave you sated.

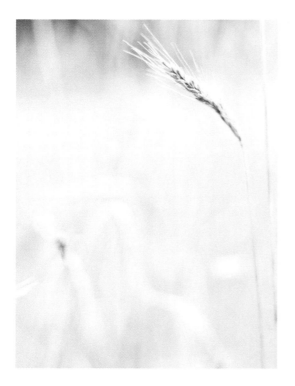
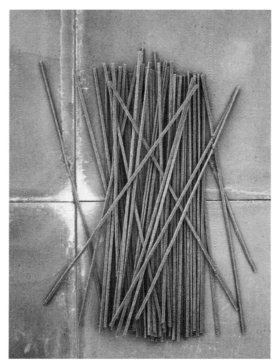
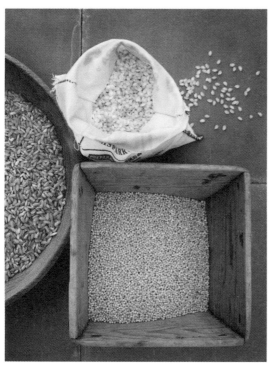
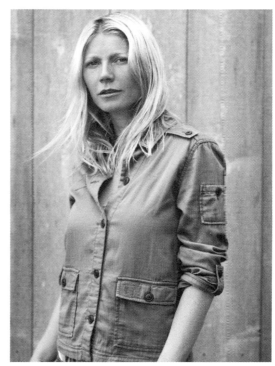

PERFECTLY COOKED QUINOA

A must for all healthy contemporary diets, quinoa is a protein-packed grain that cooks quickly and is a wonderful canvas for all sorts of add-ins and dressings. Annoyed with pot after pot of watery or overcooked quinoa, we dedicated ourselves to nailing down a fail-proof method. We now always use a less-than-two-to-one ratio of water to quinoa and tuck a paper towel between the pot and the lid while the quinoa is resting. It comes out perfect every time.

Makes 3 cups

E Elimination Diet **V** Vegan **P** Protein-Packed

1 cup quinoa
1¾ cup water
Coarse sea salt

Rinse the quinoa thoroughly in a fine-mesh strainer (although this may sound like an unnecessary step, it really makes a huge difference in flavor, since quinoa's natural coating tastes like soap).

Place it in a pot set over high heat with the water and a big pinch of salt. Bring the quinoa to a boil, lower the heat, cover the pot, and cook until all the liquid is absorbed and the quinoa's germs look like lots of little spirals, 12 to 15 minutes. Turn the heat off, place a dry paper towel between the pot and the lid, and let the quinoa sit for at least 5 minutes before giving it a fluff with a fork.

PERFECTLY COOKED BROWN RICE

It's great to keep cooked brown rice around; it's a healthy staple and you can make it in a big batch and leave it in the fridge all week. Heated up for breakfast with some rice milk and a drizzle of maple syrup or in a variety of savory dishes, brown rice is a grain I can't live without.

Makes 3 cups

E Elimination Diet **V** Vegan

1 cup short-grain brown rice
1¾ cup water
Coarse sea salt

Rinse the rice thoroughly in a fine-mesh strainer until the water runs clear.

Place it in a pot set over high heat with the water and a big pinch of salt. Bring the mixture to a boil, lower the heat, cover the pot, and cook until all the liquid is absorbed and the rice is cooked through, exactly 45 minutes. Turn the heat off, place a dry paper towel between the pot and the lid, and let the rice sit for at least 5 minutes before giving it a fluff with a fork.

SUPER-HEALTHY KOSHERI

My brother Jake's favorite side dish is kosheri (sometimes spelled koshary, kushari, or koshari), which is among the most popular street foods in Egypt. Cheap, filling, and flavorful, it's traditionally made with white rice, fried onions, lentils, and broken pieces of pasta and is often served with an oily, spicy tomato sauce. I've simplified the recipe and made it a bit healthier, too, leaving out the pasta and sauce, swapping brown rice for the white rice, and slowly cooking the onions to get tremendous flavor without buckets of oil. This is just as successful made with quinoa (simply substitute it for the brown rice and reduce the cooking time from 45 to 20 minutes). Though it requires an additional dish to clean, my absolute favorite variation is to make one pot of the brown rice version and one pot of the quinoa version and then combine them.

Serves 4

Ⓥ Vegan (made with vegetable stock)

⅓ cup lentils (preferably the dark-green French
    variety called du Puy)
Extra virgin olive oil
1 very large yellow Spanish onion (or 2 regular
    yellow onions), peeled and thinly sliced
A 2-inch cinnamon stick
4 cardamom pods, crushed with the side of
    your knife
3 whole cloves
1 cup long-grain brown rice (or quinoa)
Coarse sea salt
1¾ cups water, Vegetable Stock (see page 272),
    or Chicken Stock (see page 272)

Bring a medium pot of salted water to a boil and add the lentils. Lower the heat and simmer just until the lentils are cooked through, about 25 minutes. Drain the lentils and set them aside.

Heat ¼ cup of the olive oil in a large skillet set over medium heat. Add the onion and cook, stirring now and then, until totally soft and caramelized, a solid ½ hour. Set the onions aside.

Meanwhile, heat about 3 tablespoons of the olive oil in a large saucepan over medium heat. Add the spices and the rice or quinoa and cook the grains until they turn opaque and the spices are fragrant, about 3 minutes. Add a big pinch of salt and the water or stock. Bring to a boil, turn the heat to low, cover, and cook for 45 minutes if you're doing the brown rice version or just 20 if you're using quinoa. Turn off the heat and let the mixture sit for 10 minutes. Uncover, fluff with a fork, and fold in the lentils and onions.

RISOTTO WITH PEAS + GREENS

Risotto, usually made with tons of cheese, wine, and butter, is one of the most decadent dishes I can think of. Because Arborio rice is a beautiful grain, I wondered if I could make an equally decadent version without any of the no-no ingredients. Mission accomplished.

Serves 4

Ⓥ Vegan

1 quart Vegetable Stock (see page 272)
1 lemon
2 tablespoons extra virgin olive oil
½ yellow onion, finely diced (about ¾ cup)
1 leek, white and light green parts only,
    thoroughly washed and finely diced
2 garlic cloves, finely minced
Leaves from 6 sprigs of thyme
Coarse sea salt
1 cup Arborio rice
2 cups baby spinach or any other baby greens
    (like tatsoi)
1 cup fresh English peas (or you can substitute
    small frozen peas)
¼ cup roughly chopped fresh basil
Freshly ground black pepper

Warm the vegetable stock in a small pot and set it on the back burner over low heat.

Using a Microplane grater or a zester, zest the lemon and set the zest aside. Cut the lemon in half, juice it, and set the juice aside.

Meanwhile, heat the olive oil in a large, heavy pot set over high heat. Add the onion and leek, turn the heat down to medium, and cook until the vegetables just begin to soften, about 5 minutes. Add the garlic and thyme along with a big pinch of salt and cook until all the aromatics are, well, aromatic, another 2 minutes. Turn the heat to high, add the rice and the reserved lemon juice, and stir to combine all the ingredients. Cook until the lemon juice is just evaporated and then stir in a ladleful of the warm stock. Continue to stir the risotto until the stock is absorbed, then stir in another ladleful of stock. Continue in this manner until the rice is cooked through and you've used all your stock, about 20 minutes. At this point your arm should feel as if it's going to fall off and the rice should be luxuriously creamy and rich. Stir in the reserved lemon zest, the greens and peas (these will cook with the risotto's residual heat), the basil, and a few healthy grinds of pepper. Serve immediately.

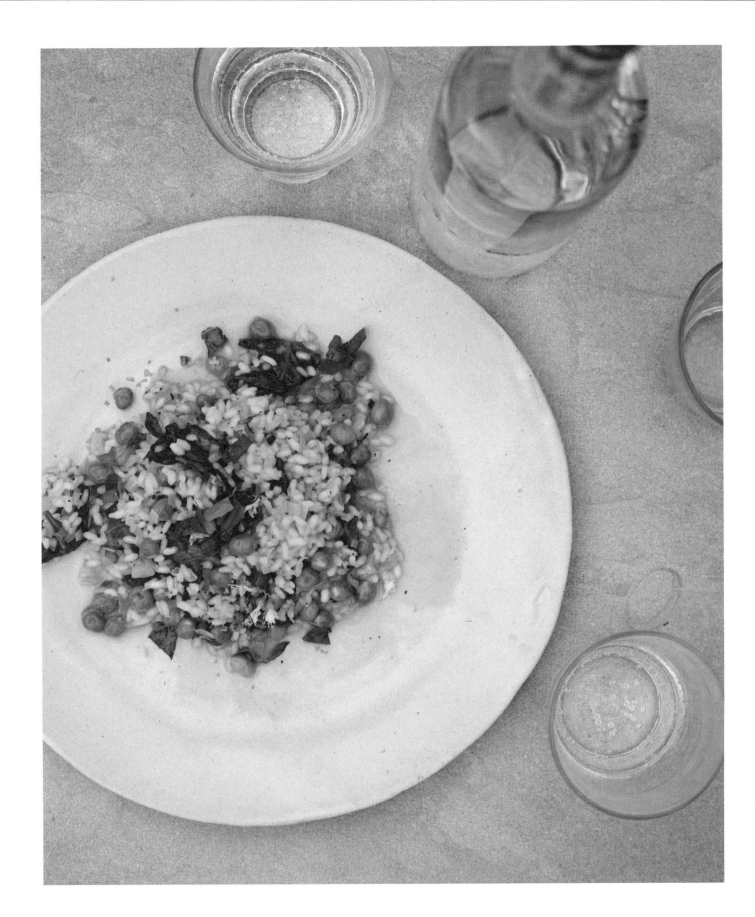

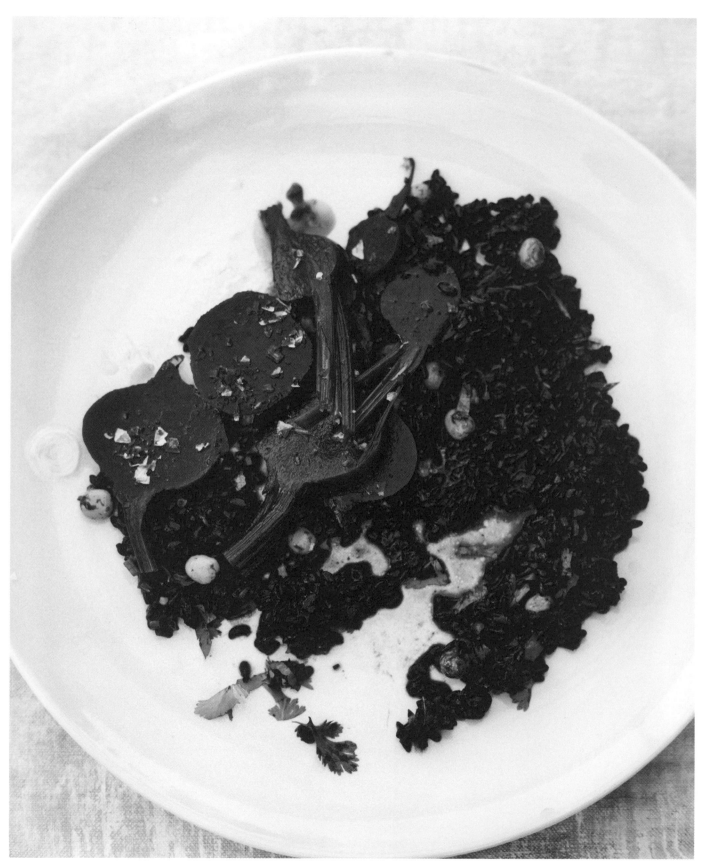

Black Rice with Fresh Coconut (opposite) served with The Simplest Beet Salad Ever (page 155)

BLACK RICE WITH FRESH COCONUT

Black rice is packed with fiber and iron and is also an antioxidant, and its nutty flavor works well with the sweetness of the coconut water. Once when I was left on a desert island during a survival course (What was I thinking?) I had only a small bag of rice and plenty of coconuts falling off of trees. That was the first time I used coconut water to make rice, and the flavor was delicious. This recipe is inspired by that little island in Belize!

Serves 4

E Elimination Diet (leave out the peas) **V** Vegan

1 fresh young coconut or 2 cups store-bought coconut water
1 cup black rice (sometimes labeled forbidden rice)
Coarse sea salt
½ cup fresh English peas (or small frozen peas)
½ cup roughly chopped cilantro
2 tablespoons roughly chopped fresh chives
1 lime

Crack open the coconut and pour the water into a measuring cup. You will need 2 cups of coconut water, so, depending on your coconut, drink a little if there's extra, or top it off with a bit of store-bought coconut water or regular water if there's not enough. Use a spoon to scrape out the soft meat from inside the coconut. Remove and discard any brown bits of shell from the coconut meat and roughly chop the meat and set it aside (the meat is optional, so don't worry if you're using store-bought coconut water).

Pour the 2 cups of coconut water into a saucepan and add the chopped coconut meat (if you've got it), the rice, and a pinch of salt. Bring the mixture to a boil, turn the heat to low, cover the pot, and simmer until the rice is cooked through, about 1 hour. Add the peas, cilantro, and chives. Finely zest the lime and add it to the rice. Cut the lime in half and squeeze the juice into the rice. Stir to combine everything and serve immediately.

MEXICAN TOMATO RICE

Along with Go-To Black Beans (see page 275), this flavorful rice is a pivotal side dish with any Mexican-inspired meal.

Serves 4

V Vegan

A 14-ounce can whole peeled tomatoes
½ yellow onion, peeled and roughly chopped
2 garlic cloves, peeled
1½ teaspoons coarse sea salt
3 tablespoons extra virgin olive oil
1 cup long-grain brown rice
3 tablespoons tomato paste
½ cup frozen peas
2 tablespoons cilantro, roughly chopped

Combine the tomatoes with the onion, garlic, and salt in a powerful blender and puree until completely smooth. Add enough water so you have 2½ cups of liquid and set it aside.

Heat the olive oil in a large, heavy saucepan set over high heat. Add the rice and cook, stirring, until the rice turns opaque and smells nutty and almost like popcorn, about 3 minutes. Stir the tomato paste into the rice and cook it for just 1 minute, so the tomato paste really gets into the rice. Add the reserved blended tomato mixture and bring the whole thing to a boil. Lower the heat, cover the pot, and simmer until the rice is cooked all the way through, about 45 minutes. Take the pot off the heat, uncover it, throw the peas on top of the rice, cover again, and let the rice sit undisturbed for 10 minutes. Remove the lid (the peas will cook from the rice's residual heat), give the whole thing a good stir, and serve sprinkled with the cilantro.

CHICKEN + TURKEY SAUSAGE PAELLA

High-quality turkey sausage is paramount for the success of this recipe. Find a sausage that is just meat, herbs, and spices, with no fillers. Organic would be even better. Browning the chicken and sausages for a super-long time creates a flavor in the pan that gives richness to the whole dish—that's always my secret.

Serves 4 generously

Ⓟ Protein-Packed

1 whole 3- to 4-pound organic chicken
6 cups Chicken Stock (see page 272)
1 teaspoon sweet pimentón
½ teaspoon hot pimentón
Coarse sea salt
Freshly ground black pepper
¼ cup extra virgin olive oil
1 pound sweet Italian turkey sausage (preferably
    freshly made, from a good butcher—not
    processed), cut into 2-inch sections
1½ yellow onions, finely diced
2 red peppers, seeds and stem removed, cut into
    1-inch pieces
4 garlic cloves, finely minced
2 medium vine-ripened tomatoes, cut in half
2 cups Bomba rice (a short-grain rice from Spain
    that's best for paella, available from La
    Tienda at www.tienda.com; or you can
    substitute Arborio rice)
A large pinch of saffron
8 small artichokes, trimmed and steamed for
    20 minutes, cut in half and the chokes
    discarded
1 cup frozen peas
2 lemons, cut into wedges

First, cut up your chicken. Remove the wings, cut off the wing tips and set them aside, and cut each wing at the joint so you're left with 4 pieces. Remove the thighs and legs in 1 piece and separate each, the left and the right, at their joints so you've got 2 drumsticks and 2 thighs. Cut each thigh in half. Remove the breasts from the carcass and cut each into 3 pieces, straight through the bone. Set aside the chicken's backbone. Alternatively, your butcher can do all this for you, but ask him or her not to discard the backbone. Or, of course, you can buy a chicken already cut into pieces.

Place the reserved backbone and the reserved wing tips in a large pot and cover with the chicken stock. Set the pot over high heat, bring to a boil, lower the heat, and simmer for 20 minutes—this will help fortify the stock and give it great...backbone. Strain the stock and return it to the stove. Stir in the sweet and hot pimentón. Salt the stock to taste (it will take a good teaspoon or so). The stock is where the rice will get all its flavor, so don't be shy with your pimentón and salt—add more of either if you think it needs it (this will depend on the salinity of your original stock). Let this flavorful mixture simmer on the back burner over the lowest possible heat while you prepare the rest of the paella.

Season the chicken pieces aggressively with salt and pepper. Heat the olive oil in a 16- to 18-inch paella pan over medium-high heat until it just begins to smoke. Add the chicken pieces, skin side down, and cook, turning now and then, until deeply browned all over and just about cooked through, a good 25 minutes (truly! don't rush the browning; it adds a crazy dimension of flavor). Remove the chicken pieces from the pan and set them aside. Add the turkey sausage pieces to the pan and, again, lovingly and patiently brown them all over, another solid 20 minutes or so. Set the sausage aside with the chicken.

Add the onions, peppers, and garlic to the pan and cook, stirring, until they're just beginning to soften, about 5 minutes. Coarsely grate in the tomatoes, discarding the skin. Stir together and cook for another 5 minutes, just to get the flavors all combined. Return the chicken and sausages to the pan along with the rice. Sprinkle the saffron over the pan, then add the stock and stir to combine everything. Bring to a boil, then lower the heat to a simmer. Arrange the artichokes and peas on top and cook until the rice is just cooked through, about 25 minutes. Remove the pan from the heat and let it sit undisturbed for 10 minutes. Serve with lemon to squeeze over the rice.

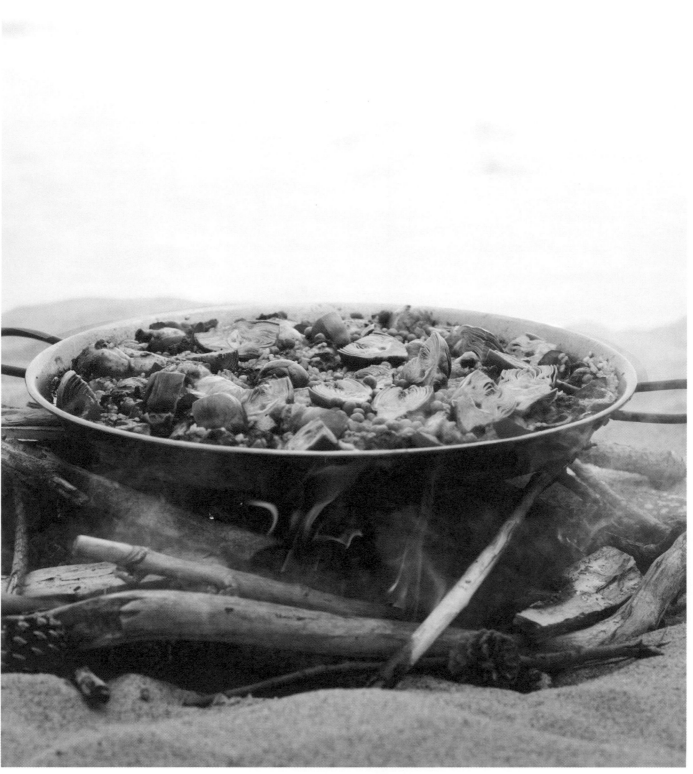

Chicken + Turkey Sausage Paella (page 184)

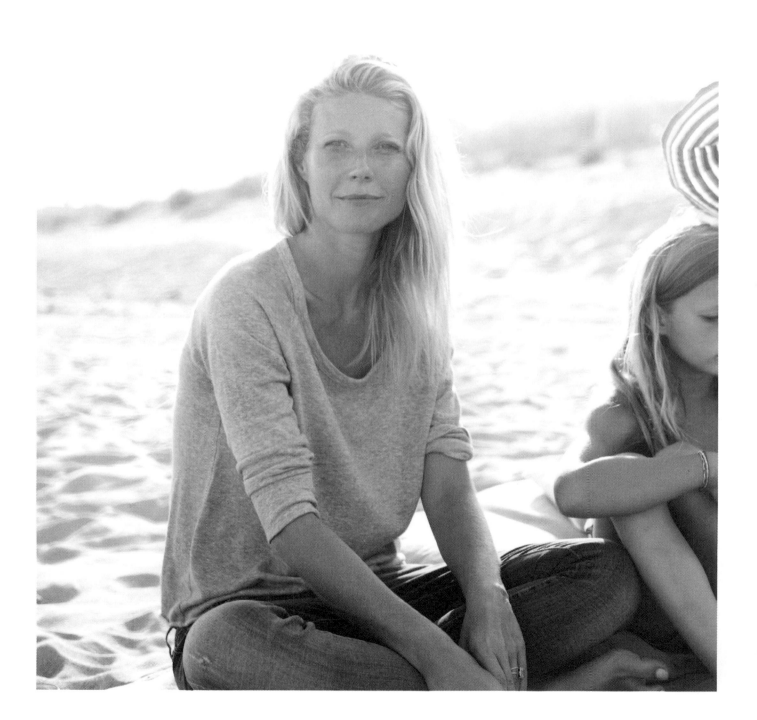

POLENTA WITH SHIITAKES + FRIED LEEKS

This beautiful dish works amazingly well as a vegetarian entrée or a side dish. Polenta is a whole grain, so it's loaded with fiber (and B vitamins, another benefit!).

Serves 4

V Vegan **P** Protein-Packed

1 small leek, thoroughly washed
Extra virgin olive oil
2 garlic cloves, finely minced
Leaves from 2 sprigs of thyme
½ pound fresh shiitake mushrooms, tough stems
    discarded, caps thinly sliced (about 3 cups)
Coarse sea salt
2½ cups Vegetable Stock (see page 272)
2 dried shiitake mushrooms
1 cup instant polenta
1 lemon

Slice the leek in half crosswise, then cut each cylinder in half lengthwise so the leek quarters can lie flat on your cutting board. Thinly slice the 4 quarters lengthwise so you have nice long, thin strands of leek. Heat about ½ inch of olive oil in a large skillet over medium-high heat and add only enough leeks that they're in a single layer (you may have to do this in batches). Cook the leeks until browned and crisp, stirring now and then, just about 2 minutes. Remove the leeks with tongs or a slotted spoon to a plate lined with a paper towel and repeat with the remaining leeks until they're all wonderfully crisp. Set the leeks aside.

Pour out most of the olive oil from the pan, leaving just a few tablespoons (reserve the extra oil for another use or discard it). Set the pan over medium-high heat and add the garlic and thyme. Cook until the aromatics begin to sizzle, but not brown, just 1 minute. Add all the fresh mushrooms (don't worry, they will shrink significantly) and stir to combine them with the garlicky oil. Cook until they get just a little bit brown, about 2 minutes. Turn the heat to low and cook for a solid ½ hour, stirring now and then, or until the mushrooms have completely softened. Salt the mushrooms to taste.

When the mushrooms are nearly done cooking, combine the stock with the dried shiitakes in a large saucepan and bring to a boil. Turn the heat to low and let the stock simmer for at least 10 minutes to get the mushroom flavor really going. Remove and discard the mushrooms, then slowly whisk in the polenta. Cook until it just comes together; it usually takes only 1 or 2 minutes, but be sure to check the directions on the box.

Stir the cooked shiitakes into the polenta and pour it onto a platter or into individual bowls. Top the polenta with the fried leeks. Finely zest half of the lemon and scatter the zest over the leeks. Give the whole thing a nice big pinch of coarse salt and serve.

SCALLION PANCAKES WITH BROWN RICE FLOUR

These addictive, super-crispy bite-sized pancakes are based on the Korean ones known as *pajeon*. You can also add chopped kimchi to the batter if you like. For a delicious dipping sauce, whisk together some soy sauce, sesame oil, and rice vinegar to taste. I can never seem to make enough of these. My family are crazy for them; they disappear in minutes!

Serves 4

Ⓥ Vegan

1 cup white spelt flour, if you can tolerate a little
    gluten, or all-purpose gluten-free flour
    (if the flour doesn't include xanthan gum,
    add ½ teaspoon)
¼ cup brown rice flour
1¼ cups ice water
1 tablespoon sesame oil
½ cup thinly sliced scallions, white and light
    green parts only
Neutral oil (like canola, grapeseed, or safflower
    oil) for frying
Coarse sea salt

Whisk the flours together with the water and sesame oil. Fold in the scallions and a large pinch of salt. Heat a shallow layer (about ¼-inch) of oil in a large nonstick pan over high heat and add as many tablespoonfuls of batter as will fit without crowding. Cook each pancake until it's nicely browned, about 2 minutes on a side. Drain the pancakes on a plate lined with a paper towel and sprinkle each with a tiny pinch of salt. Repeat the process with the remaining batter, adding more oil to the pan as needed. Serve these immediately!

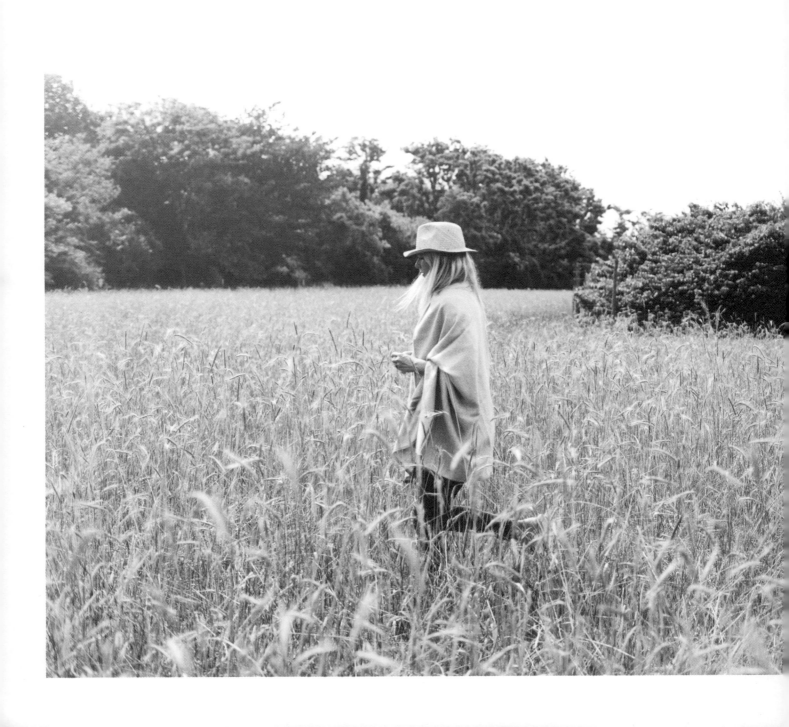

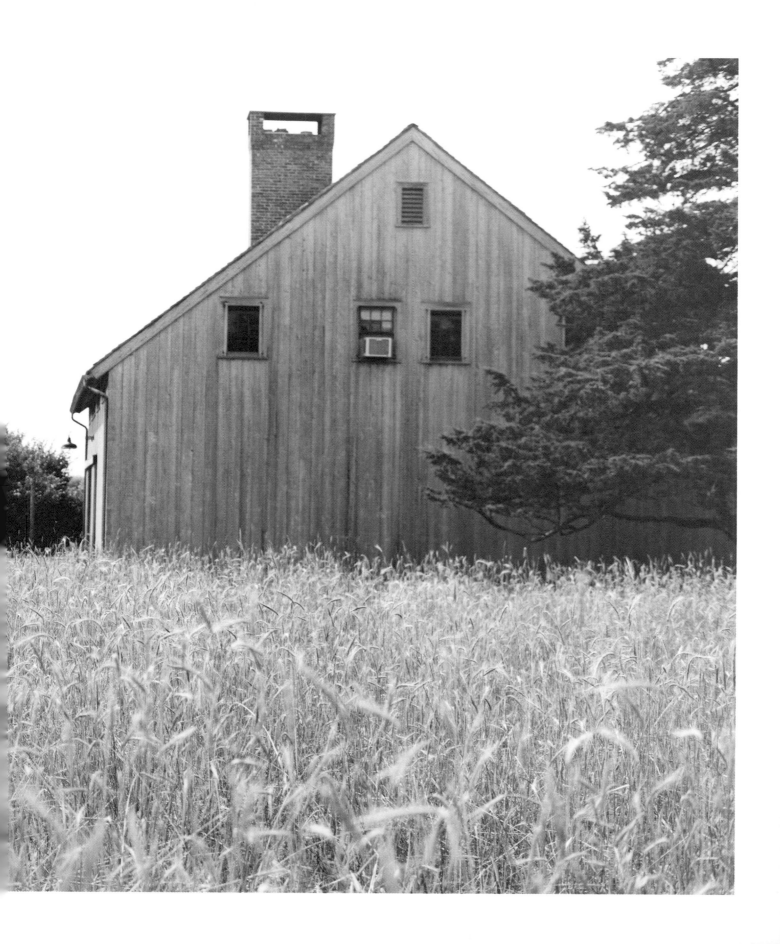

BROWN RICE PASTA WITH TUNA, OLIVES, FRIED CAPERS + PARSLEY

Brown rice pasta has many detractors, and for good reason. It doesn't stand up that well to sauces and doesn't have the same great chew as regular pasta. But when you're avoiding gluten but are dying for a bowl of pasta, it can do the trick, especially when you give it a lighter sauce, bursting with rich flavor. This recipe was inspired by a meal I had made by Gavin Rossdale (yes, he looks like that and he can cook). The result is a gorgeous entrée that seems incredibly decadent.

Serves 4

(P) Protein-Packed

8 ounces brown rice pasta (we like Lundberg
    rotini for this recipe, but whatever you're
    into)
Extra virgin olive oil
½ cup capers, rinsed and dried on a paper towel
8 garlic cloves, very thinly sliced
A dozen good-quality anchovy fillets
A big pinch of red chili flakes
A small handful of pitted Kalamata olives, split
    in half with your fingers (you want this nice
    and rustic)
16 ounces olive oil–packed tuna, oil drained off
    and discarded or saved for another use
Juice of 1 very juicy lemon
½ cup chopped Italian parsley

Bring a large pot of salted water to a boil and cook the pasta according to the package directions until just al dente.

Meanwhile, heat ½ inch of olive oil in a small skillet set over high heat and fry the capers, stirring once or twice, until really crispy, about 2 minutes (be very careful when doing this, as they tend to pop a bit).

Remove the capers from the hot oil with a slotted spoon, transfer them to a plate, and set them aside.

Heat ⅓ cup of olive oil (you can use the caper oil) in a large, heavy skillet set over medium-low heat. Add the garlic, anchovies, and chili flakes to the pan and cook, stirring constantly, until the anchovies have dissolved into the oil, the whole mixture is nice and fragrant and is softening, and the garlic is just barely beginning to brown, 3 to 4 minutes. Add the olives and tuna to the pan and stir to break up the tuna and coat everything with the nearly magical mix of garlic, anchovy, and chili. Pour the lemon juice over the mixture and stir it until it all just comes together and the tuna is warmed through and barely beginning to take on a hint of brown on its edges, 2 or 3 more minutes. Turn off the heat and add the reserved crispy capers and the parsley. At this point your pasta should be just done, drained, and ready to go.

Divide the cooked pasta among 4 serving bowls and evenly divide the tuna mixture over each portion. Serve immediately.

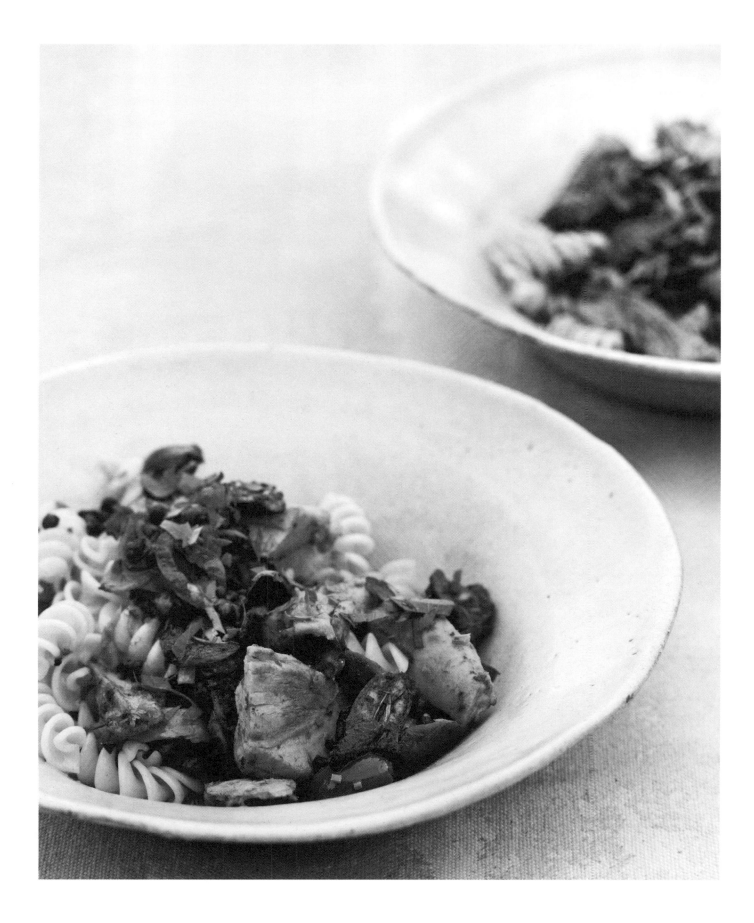

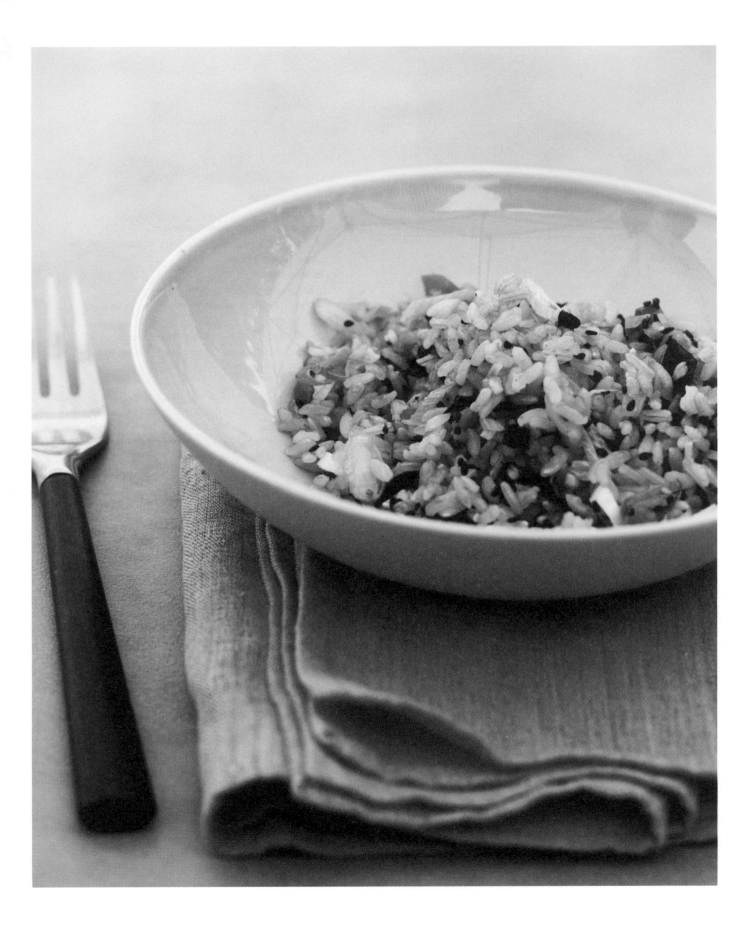

STIR-FRIED BROWN RICE WITH NORI + BLACK SESAME

This simple dish isn't just a great way to dress up leftover rice, it actually depends on leftover rice, since leftover is drier than freshly cooked rice and the kernels get browned and crispy when you stir-fry them with this lovely combination of flavors.

Serves 4

Ⓔ Elimination Diet
Ⓥ Vegan (substitute a big pinch of salt for the soy sauce)

2 tablespoons extra virgin olive oil
2 cups day-old Perfectly Cooked Brown Rice
    (see page 178)
Coarse sea salt
2 sheets toasted nori seaweed
1 teaspoon toasted sesame oil
1 teaspoon soy sauce
1 teaspoon toasted black sesame seeds
2 scallions, white and light green parts only,
    thinly sliced

Heat the olive oil in a large nonstick skillet set over high heat. Add the rice, along with a big pinch of salt, and cook, stirring, until warmed through and just barely beginning to brown, 2 to 3 minutes. Using scissors, shred the nori finely and add it along with the remaining ingredients. Stir to combine and serve immediately.

LENTIL SALAD WITH MUSTARD + TOMATOES

Just perfect. Lentils are high in protein, and this simple preparation is wonderful as a side or as a lunch main dish (you could even slip A Poached Egg on top; see page 278).

Serves 4

Ⓥ Vegan Ⓟ Protein-Packed

1 cup lentils (preferably the dark-green French
    variety called du Puy)
1 tablespoon Dijon mustard
1 tablespoon coarse seeded mustard
Juice of ½ juicy lemon
2 tablespoons white wine vinegar
¼ cup extra virgin olive oil
Coarse sea salt
1 small red onion, finely diced
1 cup halved yellow cherry tomatoes
¼ cup roughly chopped Italian parsley

Bring a large pot of salted water to a boil, add the lentils, turn the heat to medium, and cook just until the lentils are cooked through, about 20 minutes. Drain the lentils, place them in a large mixing bowl, and set them aside.

In a smaller bowl, whisk together the mustards, lemon, vinegar, olive oil, and a large pinch of salt. Add the vinaigrette to the lentils along with the onion, tomatoes, and parsley. Season the salad to taste with salt and more lemon or olive oil if you like. This salad is best if it's allowed to sit for at least ½ hour and served at room temperature.

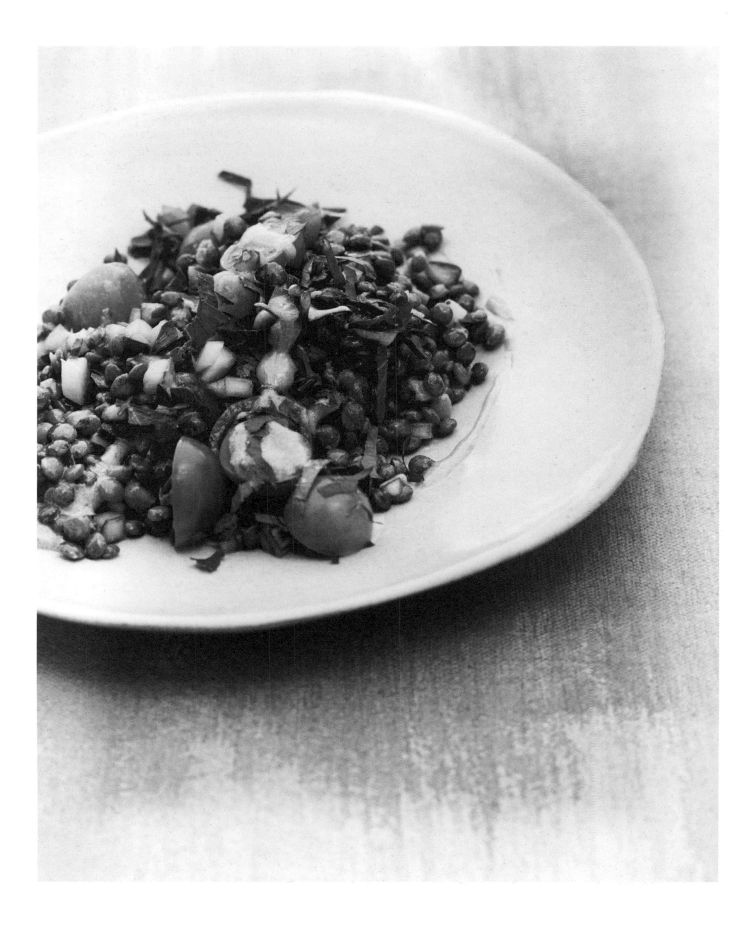

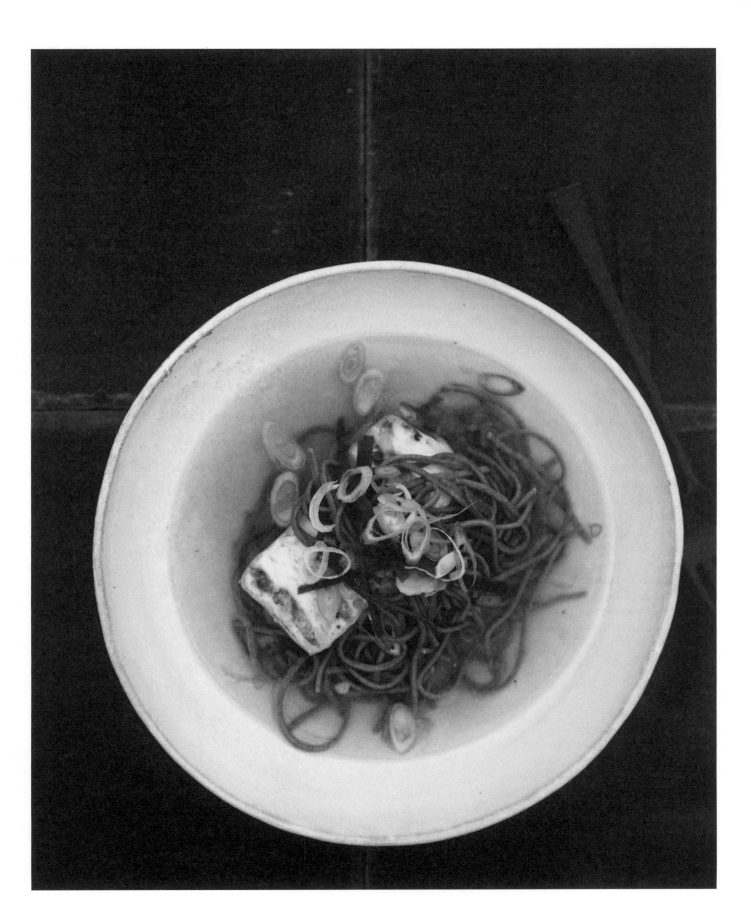

BUCKWHEAT SOBA NOODLES WITH GINGER-SCALLION BROTH

When you're skipping pasta but you really need that hearty, comforting feeling that—let's face it—only noodles can give you, buckwheat soba is the perfect trick. Buckwheat has lots of fiber and also contains all eight essential amino acids, and it will warm you up on a chilly night. If you want a bit of extra heft and a hit of protein, serve it with a few slices of grilled or broiled tofu.

Serves 4

(V) Vegan (leave out the bonito)
(P) Protein-Packed

Two 5-inch pieces of dried kombu seaweed
      (Japanese kelp), rinsed off
2 thumb-sized pieces of fresh ginger, crushed
      with the side of your knife
8 scallions, roughly chopped and bruised with
      the side of your knife, plus 2 scallions thinly
      sliced for serving
1 tablespoon plus 1 teaspoon soy sauce
2 tablespoon dried bonito flakes (leave out if
      you're vegetarian!)
8 ounces buckwheat soba noodles

Combine the kombu, ginger, chopped scallions, and soy sauce with 3 cups of cold water in a saucepan. Bring to a boil, lower the heat, add the bonito if you're using it, and simmer for 10 minutes. Strain the broth through a fine-mesh strainer into a clean pot. If you like, remove the kombu from the strainer, finely slice it, and set it aside. Discard the rest of the contents of the strainer.

Meanwhile, boil the soba noodles in a large pot of water according to the package directions. Drain the soba and divide it among 4 bowls. Evenly divide the broth among the bowls and serve topped with the thinly sliced scallions and the reserved kombu, if desired.

QUINOA WITH BUTTERNUT SQUASH, SCALLIONS + PARSLEY

This is a really beautiful way to make quinoa exciting. It's packed with flavor, freshness from the lemon, sweet earthiness from the roasted squash, and bite from the scallions...a perfect side dish.

Serves 4

E Elimination Diet **V** Vegan **P** Protein-Packed

½ butternut squash, peeled and cut into small dice (about 2 cups diced squash)
Extra virgin olive oil
Coarse sea salt
1 tablespoon freshly squeezed lemon juice
2 cups Perfectly Cooked Quinoa (page 178)
3 scallions, white and light green parts only, thinly sliced
¼ cup finely chopped Italian parsley

Preheat the oven to 400°F.

Toss the squash with 2 tablespoons of olive oil and a pinch of salt on a sheet pan and roast until soft, about 15 minutes.

Meanwhile, whisk the lemon juice with 3 tablespoons of olive oil in a large mixing bowl along with a big pinch of salt. While the squash is still warm, toss it into the dressing bowl along with the quinoa, scallions, and parsley. Taste the mixture and add a bit more salt or lemon if you feel it needs it.

QUINOA WITH MUSHROOMS + ARUGULA

This combination of earthy mushrooms and peppery arugula is another great variation on plain old quinoa.

Serves 4

E Elimination Diet **V** Vegan **P** Protein-Packed

¼ cup extra virgin olive oil
2 garlic cloves, finely minced
2 teaspoons finely chopped fresh thyme
1 pound crimini mushrooms, sliced
Coarse sea salt
2 cups Perfectly Cooked Quinoa (page 178)
2 large handfuls of arugula, roughly chopped
Freshly ground black pepper

Heat the olive oil in a large nonstick skillet set over high heat. Add the garlic and thyme to the pan and cook until they just begin to bloom and get fragrant, about 30 seconds. Add the mushrooms to the pan along with a big pinch of salt and cook, stirring now and then, until they've softened and browned and begin to make a squeaking sound (we know that sounds ridiculous, but it's true—keep your ears open). Transfer the mushroom mixture to a large mixing bowl along with the quinoa and arugula and stir to combine. Season to taste with a bit more salt and lots of freshly ground black pepper.

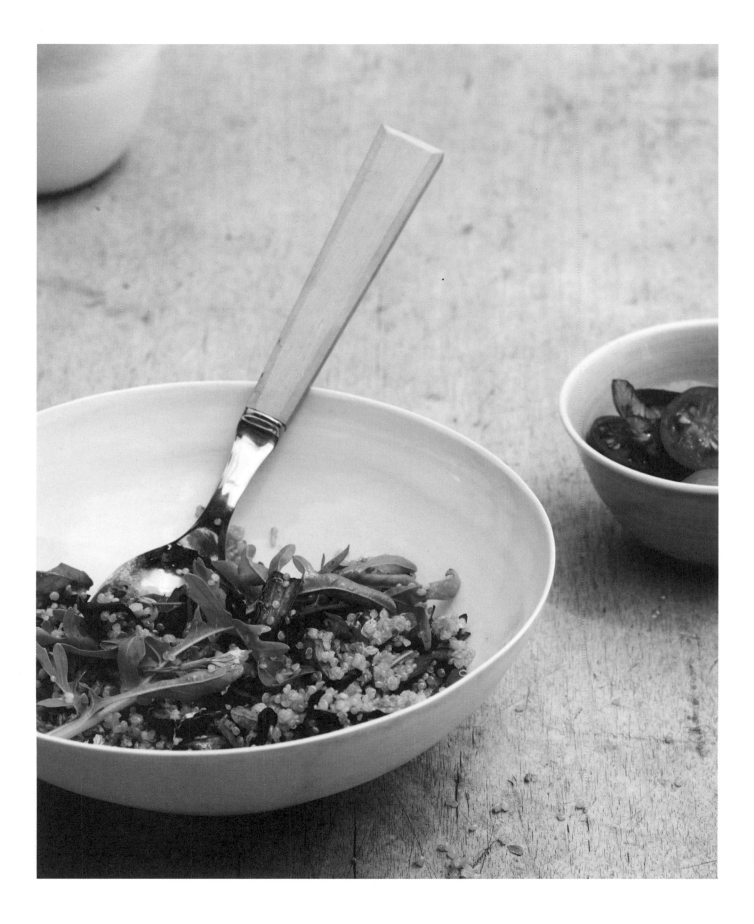

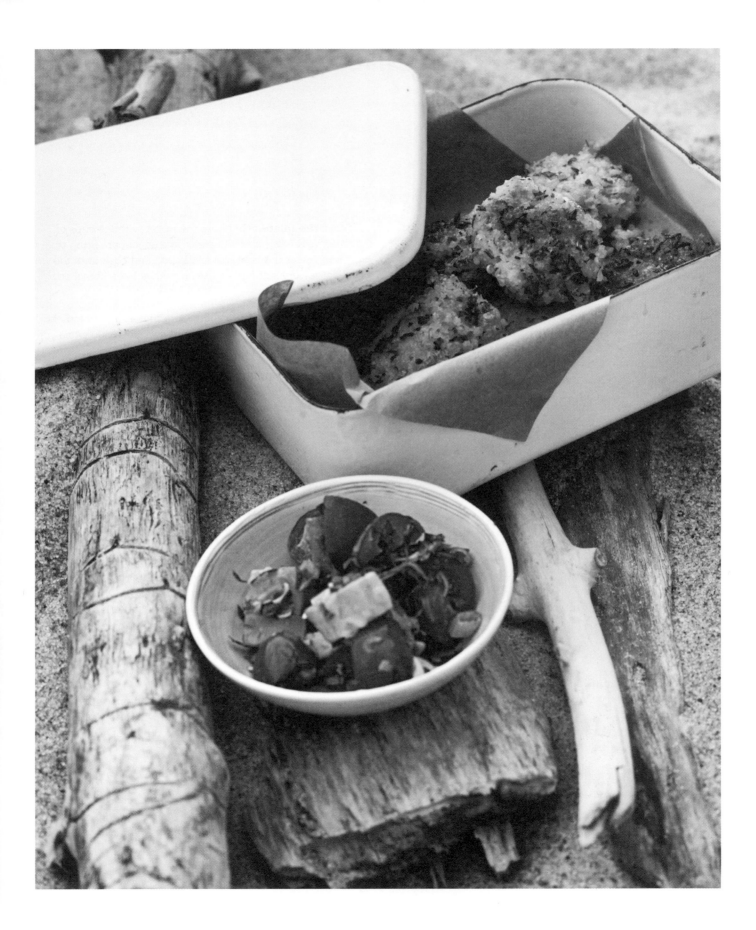

MILLET "FALAFEL" WITH AVOCADO + TOMATO RELISH

This recipe started off as a millet salad with tomatoes and scallions, but it turned into something much more interesting when we decided the salad needed a little more texture. We formed the millet into crunchy little "falafel" and mixed the tomatoes with avocado for a bright relish. Make the relish while the millet is cooking so it has a little time to settle. These are also nice with a bit of Yogurt-Tahini Dressing (see page 62).

Makes about a dozen "falafel"

E Elimination Diet (leave the tomatoes out of the relish)
V Vegan
P Protein-Packed

FOR THE FALAFEL
½ cup raw millet, rinsed
Coarse sea salt
½ cup cooked chickpeas, crushed with a potato masher
4 scallions, white and light green parts only, thinly sliced
¼ cup finely chopped Italian parsley
1 lemon
Extra virgin olive oil

FOR THE RELISH
½ cup chopped tomatoes (whatever's best; we like tiny cherry tomatoes cut in half)
1 ripe avocado, diced
2 teaspoons chopped Italian parsley
2 scallions, white and light green parts only, thinly sliced
2 teaspoons freshly squeezed lemon juice
2 tablespoons extra virgin olive oil
Coarse salt

Start the falafel: Combine the millet with 1½ cups of water and a big pinch of a salt in a saucepan. Bring to a boil, lower the heat, cover the pot, and cook until the millet is very soft and all the liquid has been absorbed, 25 minutes.

Meanwhile…for the relish: Combine all the ingredients in a bowl, seasoning to taste with salt. Set aside while you finish the falafel.

Back to the falafel…Stir the chickpeas, scallions, and parsley into the cooked millet. Using a Microplane grater, zest the lemon and stir the zest into the millet mixture along with 2 tablespoons of olive oil. Using a potato masher, crush the mixture until it holds together a bit.

Preheat the oven to 250°F and line a baking sheet with parchment paper.

Set a nonstick skillet over medium-high heat and coat the bottom with a slick of olive oil. Drop large tablespoonfuls of the millet mixture into the pan with a bit of space between each spoonful. Press each tablespoonful down with the back of a spatula to form a sort of thick pancake (no need to go crazy shaping these, they should be nice and rustic). Cook until browned and crisp, about 3 minutes per side. Set the cooked falafel on the prepared baking sheet and put them in the warm oven while you cook the rest of the millet mixture, adding more olive oil to the skillet if necessary.

Cut your zested lemon into wedges, squeeze a bit of juice over each falafel, and sprinkle each with a tiny pinch of coarse salt. Put a spoonful of relish on top of each falafel and serve immediately.

SOME DRINKS

When you're trying to get healthier and cutting out sugar, drinks can help you find that lovely sweetness you're searching for after a meal. A beautiful *agua fresca,* a hot ginger tea, a fresh juice, or an afternoon smoothie can be the perfect way to give in to those sugar cravings without actually giving in to them.

For a super-healthy and delicious way to start the day, a smoothie is a great choice, especially for someone like me who doesn't have a big appetite in the morning. For a long while, Julia and I have been fans of good protein powders for an extra boost. But our docs recommend a mix of proteins and say you shouldn't have the same thing every day anyway. So in addition to the more traditional "protein" smoothie, we've also devised some beautiful smoothies that don't have any processed powders. Enjoy!

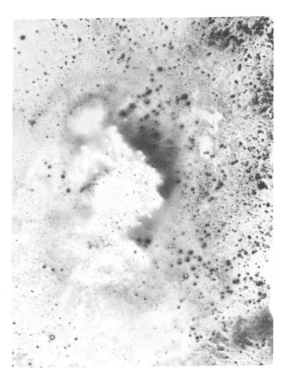
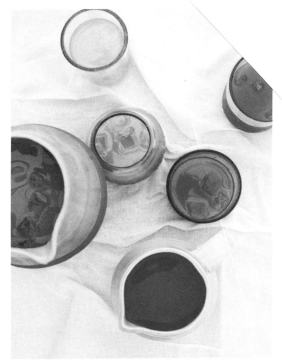
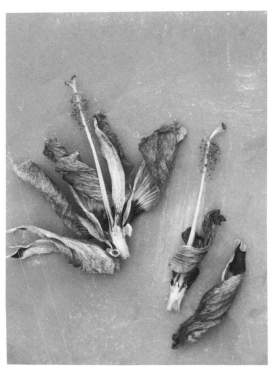
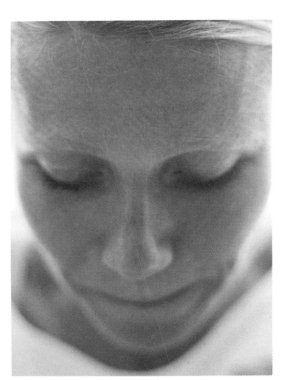

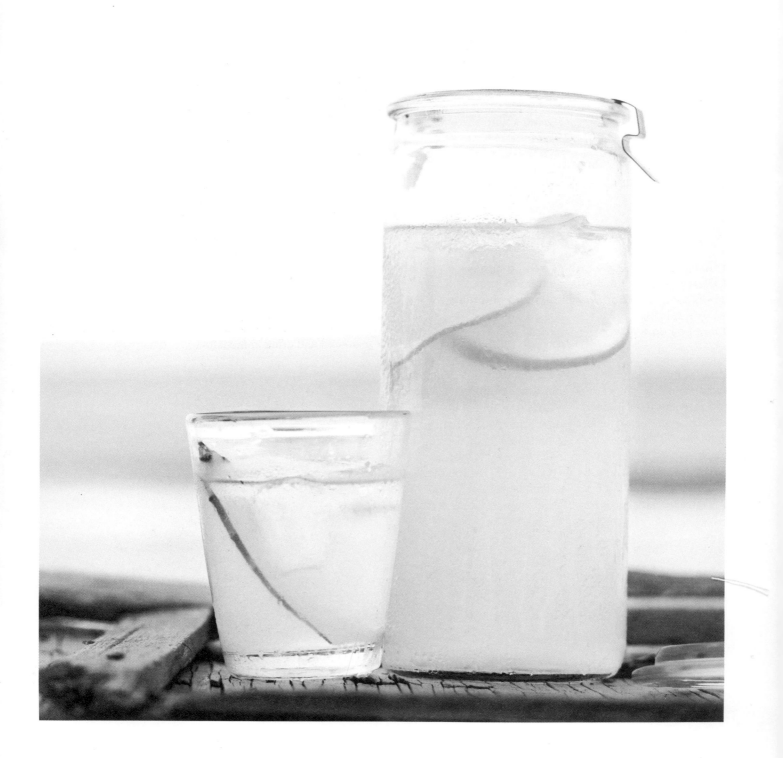

FRESH GINGER TEA

Ginger is detoxifying and warming and packs a serious flavor punch. This tea is perfect if you're trying to stay away from coffee but want a hot drink with some real depth. Terrific for colds or irritated vocal cords or as a digestive, this multipurpose tea is always brewing at my house. For a refreshing cool version, strain the mixture and serve it over plenty of ice.

Serves 1

V Vegan

1 teaspoon very finely grated fresh ginger
1 tablespoon freshly squeezed lemon juice
2 teaspoons raw honey, xylitol, or good-quality
    maple syrup
1 cup boiling water

Combine all the ingredients in a teacup or small pitcher, stir to combine, and let it sit for 2 minutes. If you want to avoid the bits of ginger fiber, pour the tea through a fine-mesh strainer into a clean teacup. And feel free to adjust the amounts to your liking—some people want their ginger tea to be tart like lemonade; others like the ginger to really blast through their sinuses; kids like it sweet—whatever works. Serve immediately, or you can also make this in a big batch and reheat it through the day (or, alternatively, pour servings over tall glasses of ice).

ALMOND + KALE SMOOTHIE

This might sound like a bummer, but it's incredibly delicious and absolutely packed with nutrition.

Serves 1 generously

E Elimination Diet **V** Vegan **P** Protein-Packed

1 packed cup torn kale leaves (discard the thick
    rib in the center of the leaf)
1 cup unsweetened almond milk
1 tablespoon almond butter
1 tablespoon Soaked Raw Almonds
    (see page 277)
1 date, pitted
1 tablespoon coconut oil

Blend everything in a powerful blender until completely smooth and drink immediately.

RED SMOOTHIE

I soaked goji berries overnight (see Soaked Goji Berries, page 277) until they became plump and added them to other berries and yogurt for a winning combination of superfoods.

Serves 1 generously

1 large spoonful goji berries, soaked in water
    overnight and drained
¼ cup fresh raspberries
3 large strawberries, stems discarded
1 tablespoon manuka honey
3 tablespoons goat's milk yogurt
1 tablespoon coconut oil
1 cup unsweetened almond milk

Blend everything together in a powerful blender until completely smooth and drink

CREAMY AVOCADO + CACAO SMOOTHIE

I first got the idea of putting avocados in smoothies from Dr. Frank Lipman of the Eleven Eleven Wellness Center in New York City. His ingenious plan to use avocado as the base makes drinks creamy and sumptuous. Here we add cacao powder and hempseeds, two superfoods, and the result is a breakfast smoothie that tastes so beautiful you won't believe it's so good for you.

Serves 2

Ⓔ Elimination Diet (leave out the honey)
Ⓥ Vegan
Ⓟ Protein-Packed

1 ripe avocado, peeled and pitted
1 cup fresh coconut water
1 cup cold unsweetened almond milk
1 tablespoon raw cacao powder
1 heaping tablespoon ground hempseeds
1 tablespoon raw honey

Blend everything in a powerful blender until completely smooth and drink immediately.

BERNARDO'S PUMPKIN PIE SHAKE

We know a trainer named Bernardo who invented a smoothie for his clients that is amazing. We tweaked it here and there and created our own version, which tastes just like pumpkin pie. I gave it to my trainer, Tracy Anderson, and she was thrilled with it. She has a big sweet tooth but said it took away her cravings for candy. Also, cloves are anti-inflammatory, nutmeg is antibacterial, and both contain eugenol, which they say benefits the heart. Thank you, Bernardo!

Serves 1

E Elimination Diet
V Vegan (use vegan protein powder)
P Protein-Packed

⅔ cup roasted sweet potato (flesh from ½ roasted sweet potato)
1½ cups cold unsweetened vanilla-flavored almond milk
1 serving whey protein powder
¼ teaspoon each ground cloves, ground ginger, and ground nutmeg
1 date, pitted
½ cup ice cubes

Blend everything in a powerful blender and drink immediately.

BODY BUILDER SMOOTHIE

Packed with vitamins and minerals from the greens powder, made sweet with a date and creamy with almond milk and banana, this super-high-protein shake will set you up for your day or workout and is also a great recovery beverage to enjoy right after your workout.

Serves 1

V Vegan (use vegan protein powder)
P Protein-Packed

1 serving whey protein powder
1 serving greens powder (a variety of brands are available at Whole Foods and health food stores)
1½ cups cold unsweetened vanilla-flavored almond milk
1 date, pitted
⅓ banana

Blend everything in a powerful blender and drink immediately.

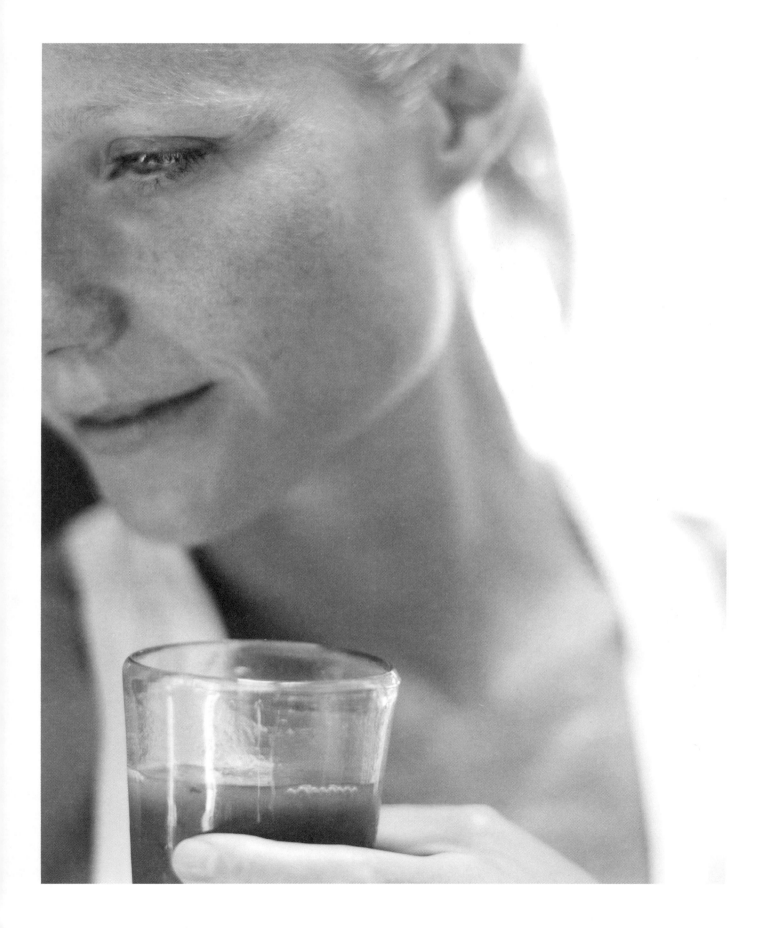

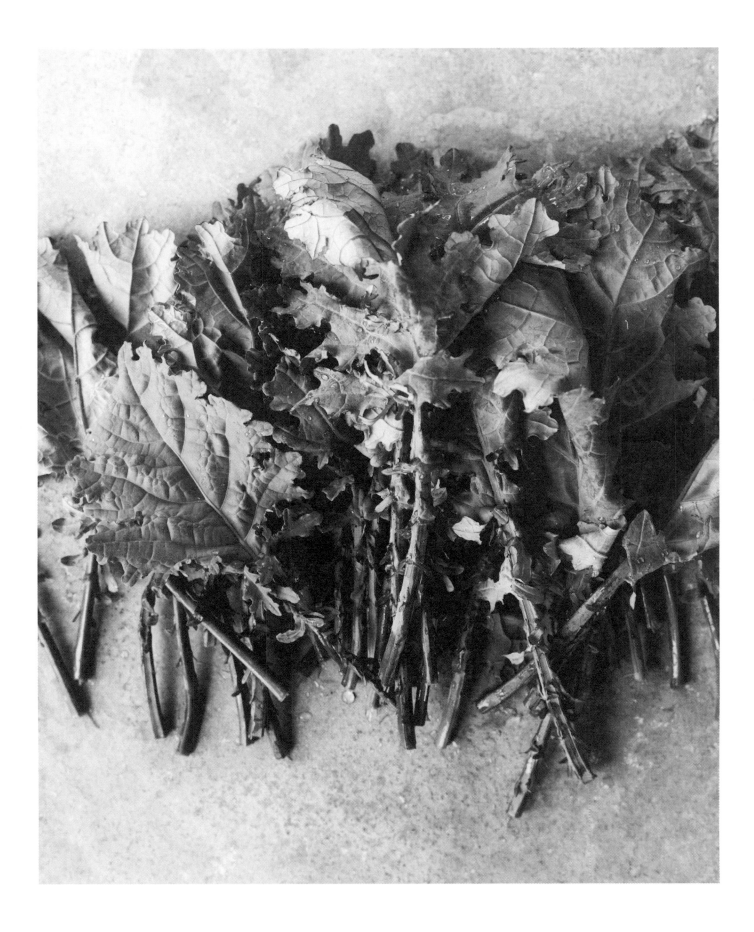

THE BEST GREEN JUICE

Just about as energizing as a cup of coffee with none of the letdown, green juice is an incredibly healthy, invigorating way to start your day. Kale is full of calcium and antioxidants and just about everything else—it's one of the best things you can put into your system. When juiced with a bit of lemon, apple, and ginger and a tiny hit of refreshing mint, it turns into a sort-of grassy lemonade. No worries if you don't have a juicer—a blender and a strainer do the trick.

Serves 1

E Elimination Diet **V** Vegan

5 large leaves of kale, ribs discarded, leaves
    roughly chopped
1 lemon, zest and pith removed
1 large apple, roughly chopped
A 1-inch piece of fresh ginger
1 sprig of fresh mint

Push all the ingredients through your juicer. Alternatively, you can chop all the ingredients and pop them into a powerful blender with ½ cup of water, then pass the mixture through a fine-mesh strainer and drink immediately.

BEET, CARROT, APPLE + GINGER JUICE

This juice is the most incredible color and is wonderfully sweet. Beets are said to lower blood pressure, carrots pack a super beta-carotene punch, apples are cancer fighters, and ginger just loves your heart.

Serves 1

E Elimination Diet **V** Vegan

1 large or 2 medium beets, cut into wedges
2 large carrots
1 large apple, cut into wedges
A 1-inch piece of fresh ginger
½ lemon, zest and pith removed

Juice everything into a glass. Alternatively, you can finely chop all the ingredients and pop them into a powerful blender with ½ cup of water, then pass the mixture through a fine-mesh strainer into a glass. Stir and drink immediately.

CUCUMBER, BASIL + LIME JUICE

This juice is especially refreshing when you blend it with a handful of ice cubes (use a whole lime if you do, as the acid is muted when the juice is cold). Think of it as a detox-friendly mojito.

Serves 1

E Elimination Diet **V** Vegan

½ cup basil leaves
1 English cucumber, cut in half lengthwise
½ lime, zest and pith removed
1 apple, cut into wedges

Starting with the basil, juice everything into a glass. Alternatively, you can chop all the ingredients and pop them into a powerful blender with ½ cup of water, then pass the mixture through a fine-mesh strainer into a glass. Give it a stir and drink immediately.

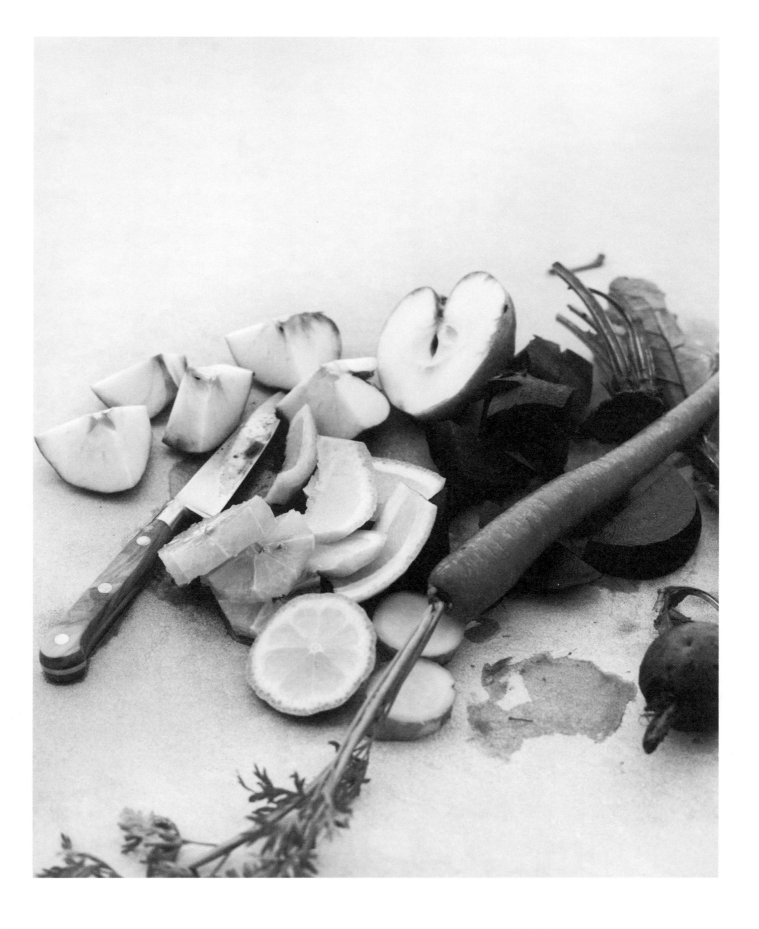

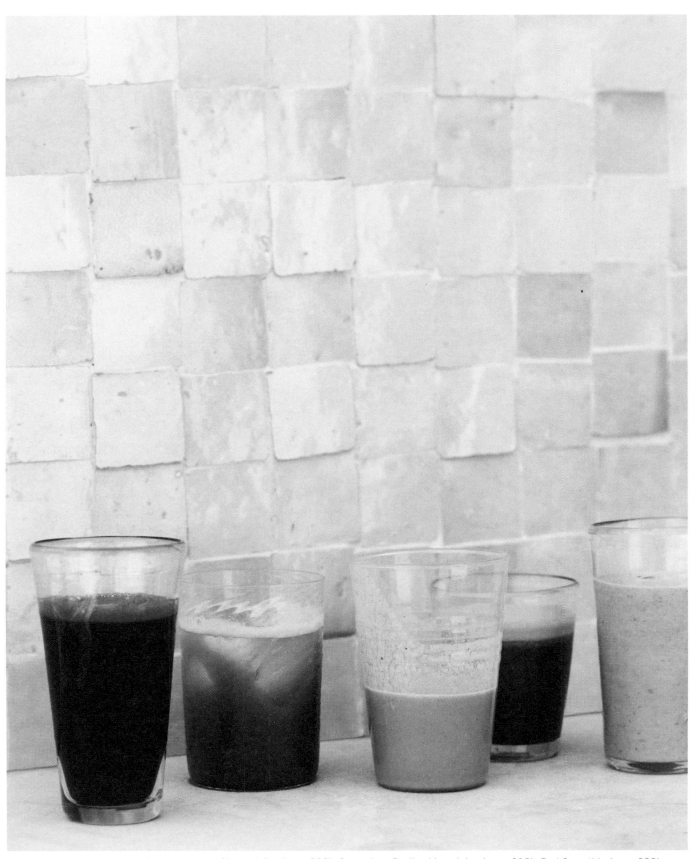

From left to right, Beet, Carrot, Apple + Ginger Juice (page 213); Cucumber, Basil + Lime Juice (page 213); Red Smoothie (page 208); The Best Green Juice (page 212); Almond + Kale Smoothie (page 207)

SUSIE'S AGUAS FRESCAS

My dear friend and beloved food stylist Susie Theodorou (this book would look like nothing without her) came to the rescue when we were discussing how to make our *aguas frescas*. She developed a brilliant, simple honey syrup that's at the base of each version and then, seemingly with tremendous ease, came up with beautiful flavor combinations. You can try whatever fruit and pairings you like, using the ratios as a guide, and can always add a bit more water or ice to any of the drinks if they taste too sweet for you. And, of course, you can add more honey if they're not sweet enough for your palate. We think they're just right.

WATERMELON + MINT

Makes about 2 quarts

Ⓥ Vegan

3 cups water
½ cup raw honey
1 small bunch of mint
1 small seedless watermelon, peeled and
    cut into cubes (about 10 cups)

Combine the water, honey, and mint in a saucepan and bring to a boil. Pull out the mint and discard it (otherwise the syrup will go bitter) and let the syrup cool to room temperature.

While the syrup is cooling, puree the watermelon, in batches, in a food processor or a blender, then pass the mixture through a fine-mesh strainer and discard the contents of the strainer. Combine the watermelon juice and the honey syrup in a pitcher, stir, and serve over ice. Drink immediately or store in the fridge for up to a day (you want the flavors to be nice and fresh). A piece of lime or grapefruit added to this drink wouldn't be bad, either.

PEAR + LEMON VERBENA

Makes about 2 quarts

Ⓥ Vegan

3 cups water
½ cup raw honey
2½ pounds pears (about 6 pears), stemmed
    and seeded and cut into large pieces
1 sprig of leafy lemon verbena
Juice of 2 lemons

Combine the water, honey, pears, and lemon verbena in a large pot set over high heat. Bring to a boil, turn off the heat, remove and discard the lemon verbena, and cover the pot. Let the mixture cool to room temperature. Puree the mixture in a powerful blender in batches and pass the puree through a fine-mesh strainer or a sieve lined with cheesecloth. Discard the contents of the strainer and whisk the lemon juice into the *agua fresca*. Serve immediately over ice.

PAPAYA + LIME

Makes about 2 quarts

Ⓥ Vegan

3 cups water
½ cup raw honey
3 pounds papaya (1 very large papaya or
    2 regular ones), peeled, seeded, and
    cut into large pieces
Juice of 2 limes

Combine the water, honey, and papaya in a large pot
set over high heat. Bring to a boil and turn off the heat.
Let the mixture cool to room temperature. Puree the
mixture in a powerful blender in batches and pass the
puree through a fine-mesh strainer or a sieve lined
with cheesecloth. Discard the contents of the strainer
and whisk the lime juice into the *agua fresca*. Serve
immediately over ice.

WHITE PEACH + GINGER

Makes about 2 quarts

Ⓥ Vegan

3 cups water
½ cup raw honey
2½ pounds white peaches (about 8 peaches),
    pits discarded, roughly chopped
A 2-inch knob of fresh ginger, peeled and sliced

Combine all the ingredients in a large pot set over high
heat. Bring to a boil, turn off the heat, and cover the pot.
Let the mixture cool to room temperature. Puree in a
powerful blender in batches and pass the puree through
a fine-mesh strainer or a sieve lined with cheesecloth.
Discard the contents of the strainer and serve the *agua
fresca* immediately over ice.

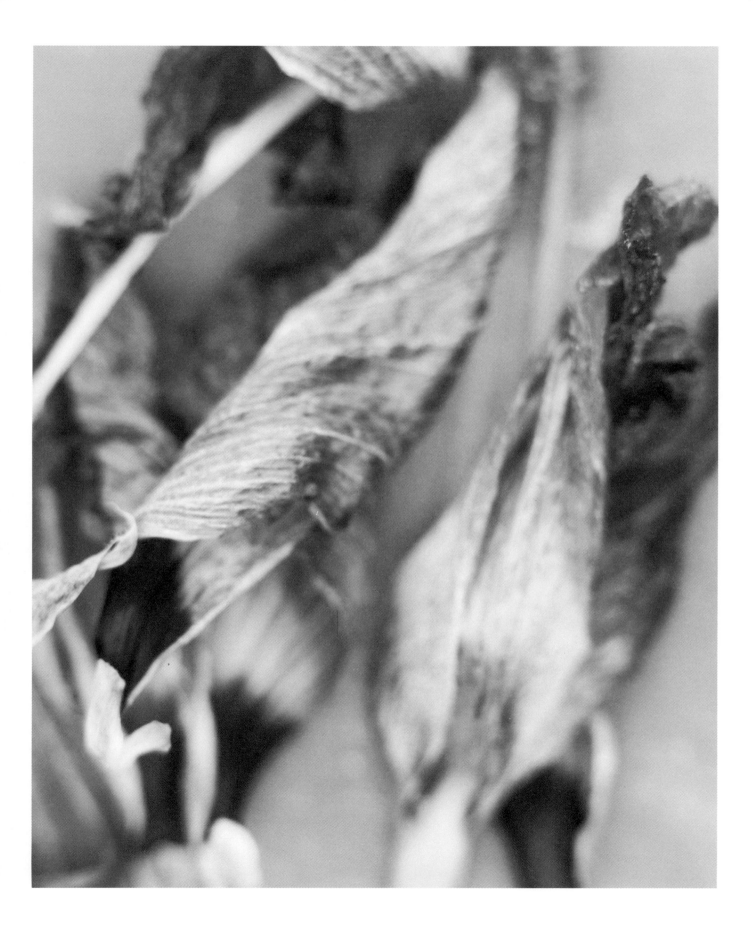

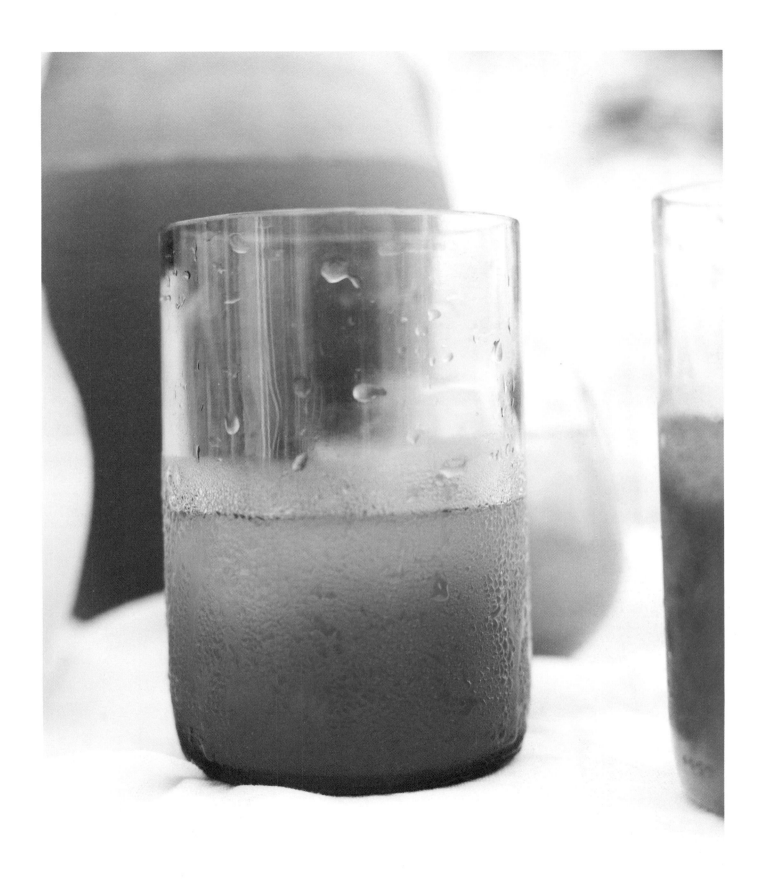

Papaya + Lime Agua Fresca (page 217)

CLEO'S AFTERNOON SHAKE

My old assistant, Cleo, insisted we include her secret afternoon shake. She drinks it around three or four o'clock for a healthy dose of protein to get her through the rest of the day. It's delicious.

Serves 1

V Vegan **P** Protein-Packed

½ ripe banana (preferably frozen)
1 tablespoon almond butter
1 date, pitted
¾ cup cold unsweetened almond milk

Combine all the ingredients in a powerful blender and blitz until smooth. Pour into a glass and enjoy immediately.

HOMEMADE ALMOND MILK/HORCHATA

Serves 1

E Elimination Diet **V** Vegan **P** Protein-Packed

For each serving, place ½ cup of Soaked Raw Almonds (see page 277) in a powerful blender. Add cold water to cover the almonds and blend until completely pureed. Pass the mixture through a fine-mesh strainer into a bowl or pitcher. Drink immediately, or keep it covered in the fridge for up to 3 days.

For *horchata* (our version of the traditional Mexican drink), return the strained almond milk to the blender along with a generous pinch of salt, the seeds of a vanilla bean, and as much raw honey as you like (I like 1 spoonful per serving).

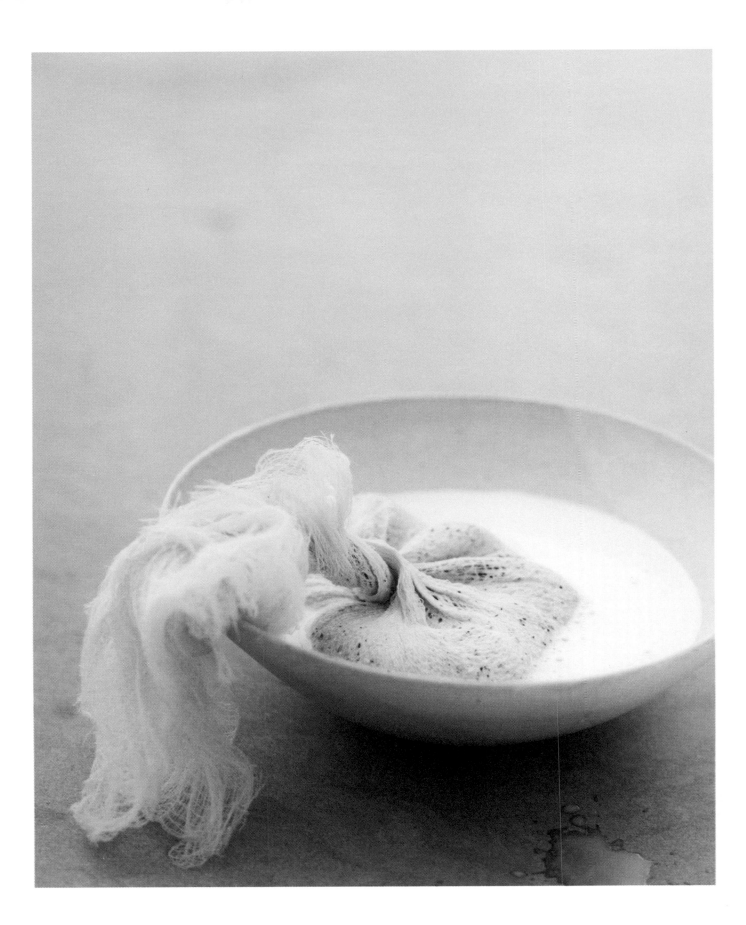

THE KIDS' MENU

Cooking with and for kids can be, as any home cook knows, a lot more complex than it looks. One week they love something, the next week they go totally off it. New foods are alternately interesting and terrifying. Over the years, I have figured out a few tricks that keep my kids engaged, enthusiastic, and, above all, eating (something that has become even more challenging now that we're trying to avoid gluten, cow's milk, etc.). I keep flavors pretty simple, don't introduce more than one new thing in any one meal, serve it small (mini-meatballs, mini-burgers, mini–shepherd's pies, etc.), serve things on a stick, and of course…with dipping sauce! The more I learn about nutrition and overall health, the more urgent it feels to feed kids the things they really need and to avoid the things that may compromise them, especially if they have allergies, eczema (like my son), or any condition at all that is exacerbated by too much white flour, ice cream, and sugar. Their health and happiness are paramount—and sometimes, when it comes to food, health and happiness can seem mutually exclusive. Here Julia and I have created a kids' chapter that we hope bridges that gap, with recipes that are kid-friendly, easy, and totally good for them.

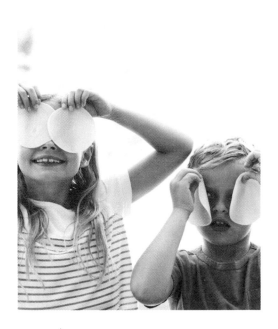
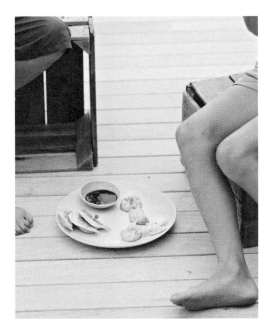
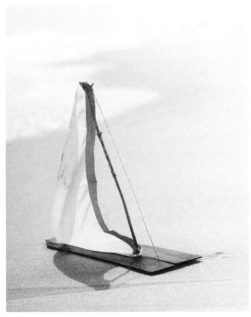
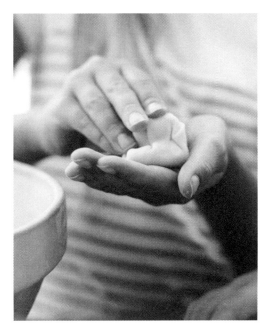

KID SMOOTHIE

Smoothies are an excellent way to get nutrients into kids. I am partial to simple smoothies based around Ultracare for Kids. It's a rice protein powder made by Metagenics; it provides tons of calcium without dairy, is completely vegan and gluten free, and is especially good for atopic problems like eczema and asthma. My kids love the vanilla flavor and ask for it regularly. They call it the healthy vanilla shake.

Serves 1

E Elimination Diet **V** Vegan **P** Protein-Packed

1 serving Ultracare for Kids or your favorite kid-friendly nutritional supplement
1 cup cold unsweetened rice or almond milk
Optional: a handful of fresh or frozen blueberries, a spoonful of raw cacao powder, or a spoonful of Soaked Goji Berries (see page 277)

Combine the supplement and the rice or almond milk in a powerful blender. Add one of the optional mix-ins if your kid is partial to any of them! Blend, then serve.

MOMO'S SPECIAL TURKEY BACON

My son, Moses, loves being in the kitchen, cooking and coming up with interesting flavors. He thought up this winning combination because he likes to dip his turkey bacon in a mustard-maple mix. We decided to use it as a sort-of shellac on the bacon, and it is delicious.

Serves 4

P Protein-Packed

An 8-ounce pack turkey bacon (usually 8 slices), cooked
2 tablespoons yellow mustard
2 tablespoons good-quality maple syrup

Preheat the broiler.

Lay the bacon on a foil-lined cookie sheet. Whisk together the mustard and maple syrup and "paint" half of it on the slices with a spoon or a pastry brush. Broil for 1 minute, then turn it and coat the other side of each slice with the remaining mixture. Broil for another 1 or 2 minutes, or until crispy and lacquered, then serve immediately.

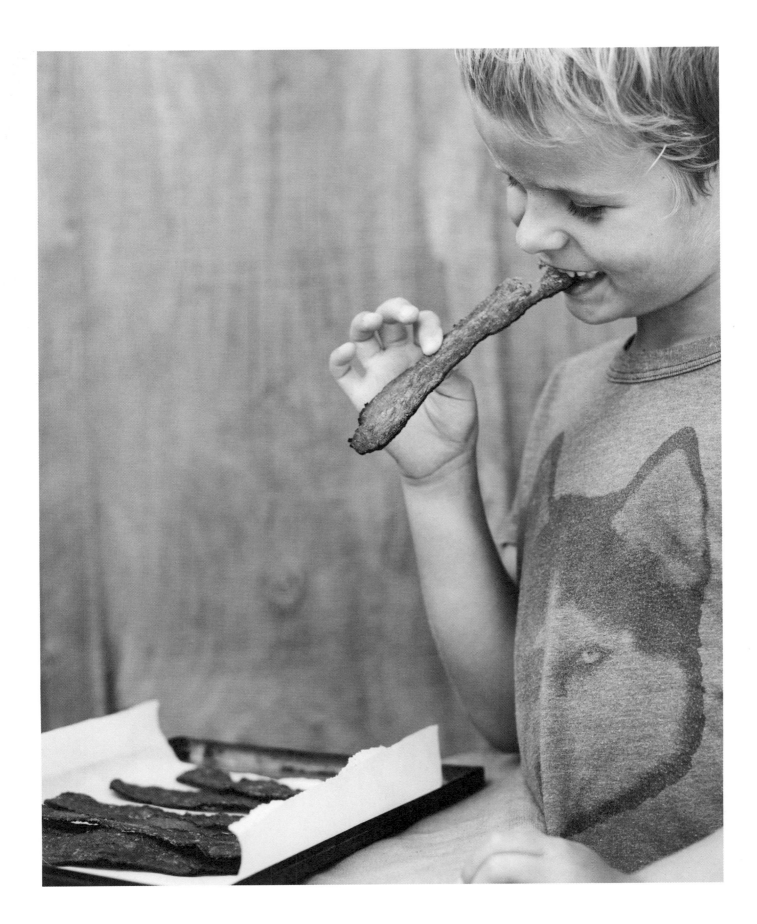

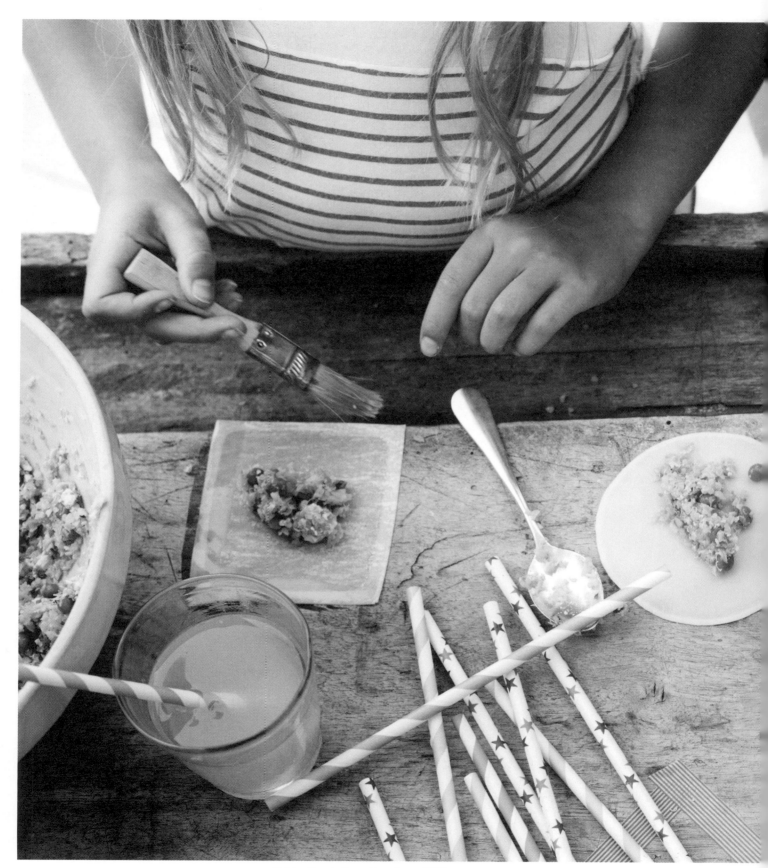

Making Veggie Dumplings (page 228)

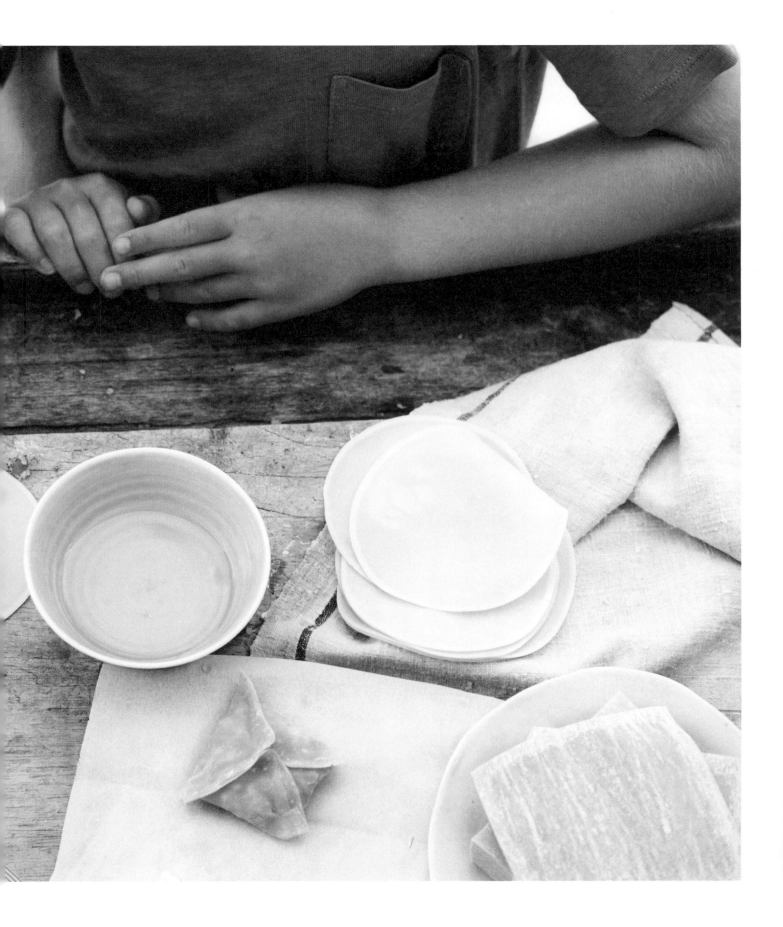

VEGGIE DUMPLINGS

These veggie dumplings make me and my kids so happy. They are packed with nutrients and are the perfect finger food. They're completely vegan and completely delicious, fun, and easy to make. You can prepare them in batches and keep them in the freezer for a wonderful family/kid dinner.

Note: To freeze the uncooked dumplings so they don't stick together, line them up on a sheet tray and stick them in the freezer. Once they're frozen, remove the tray from the freezer and pop the individual dumplings into an airtight container or zip-top plastic bag. They can be steamed or pan-fried right from the freezer, without defrosting.

Makes 30 dumplings

Ⓥ Vegan Ⓟ Protein-Packed

½ small red or yellow onion, roughly chopped
1 garlic clove, crushed
1½ cups roughly chopped Savoy or green
    cabbage
Neutral oil (like canola, grapeseed, or safflower
    oil)
Coarse sea salt
½ cup crumbled firm tofu
½ cup frozen peas
½ cup Perfectly Cooked Quinoa (page 178)
1 tablespoon soy sauce
½ teaspoon toasted sesame oil
30 square dumpling wrappers (see the recipe
    on page 229 for Homemade Gluten-Free
    Dumpling Wrappers, or find premade ones
    near the tofu in the refrigerator section of
    the grocery store—we know they're usually
    made with wheat, but considering that
    they're a vehicle for quinoa and veggies,
    we're pretty okay letting a little gluten fly
    here!)
Dipping Sauce, for serving

Blitz the onion, garlic, and cabbage together in a food processor until finely chopped. Heat 2 tablespoons neutral oil over medium-high heat in a large nonstick skillet and add the cabbage mixture and a large pinch of salt. Cook, stirring now and then, until the vegetables have softened and are just beginning to brown, 5 to 6 minutes. Stir in the tofu, peas, and quinoa and cook until the peas are totally soft, 2 to 3 minutes. Turn off the heat and add the soy sauce and sesame oil. Using a potato masher, crush the mixture so it just begins to hold together. Let the mixture cool to room temperature.

Lay a few of your dumpling wrappers on a flat, dry surface and put 1 tablespoon of filling mixture in the middle of each wrapper. Dip your index finger in a little bowl of water and use it to "paint" the edges of each dumpling. Bring each edge together to form a sort-of little pyramid (see the photos on pages 226 and 227), being sure to press all the edges to form a tight seal.

To cook, use a bamboo steamer set over simmering water to steam the dumplings for 4 minutes. Or you can do them Chinese restaurant style (a combo of frying and steaming) by heating a slick of neutral oil in a large nonstick pan set over high heat and cooking the dumplings for 2 minutes, or until they're golden brown on the bottom. Then add ½ cup of water to the pan (it will create a lot of steam, so stand back), put a lid on it, and let the dumplings steam until the wrappers are totally soft, another 2 minutes. Remove from the pan and serve with the Dipping Sauce.

DIPPING SAUCE

Ⓥ Vegan

3 tablespoons soy sauce
2 tablespoons water
1 tablespoon freshly squeezed lemon juice
1 teaspoon toasted sesame oil

Mix all the ingredients together, adding more of any of them if you prefer the sauce saltier, or more tart, or milder—it's a real throw-it-together, not-exact thing.

HOMEMADE GLUTEN-FREE DUMPLING WRAPPERS

Makes 30 dumpling wrappers

Ⓥ Vegan

3 cups all-purpose gluten-free baking flour
2¼ cups boiling water

Place the flour in a large bowl and make a well in the center. Carefully pour in the water and stir together with a spoon. Continue mixing with the spoon until a dough begins to form (it will look as if you need more water, but don't add any!) and the mixture is cool enough to handle. Ditch the spoon and knead the dough in the bowl with your hands until all the flour is absorbed and a smooth dough begins to form. Line a portion of your kitchen counter with a sheet of parchment paper and turn the dough out onto it. Continue to knead for 1 more minute, until the dough is very smooth. Cut the dough into 30 equal portions. Cover all but 1 with an ever-so-damp kitchen towel. With a rolling pin (or a wine bottle!), roll the lonely piece until it's a flat 4-inch-wide circle. Fill your rolled-out wrappers 1 at a time as in the dumpling recipe above, keeping the others covered with the damp towel.

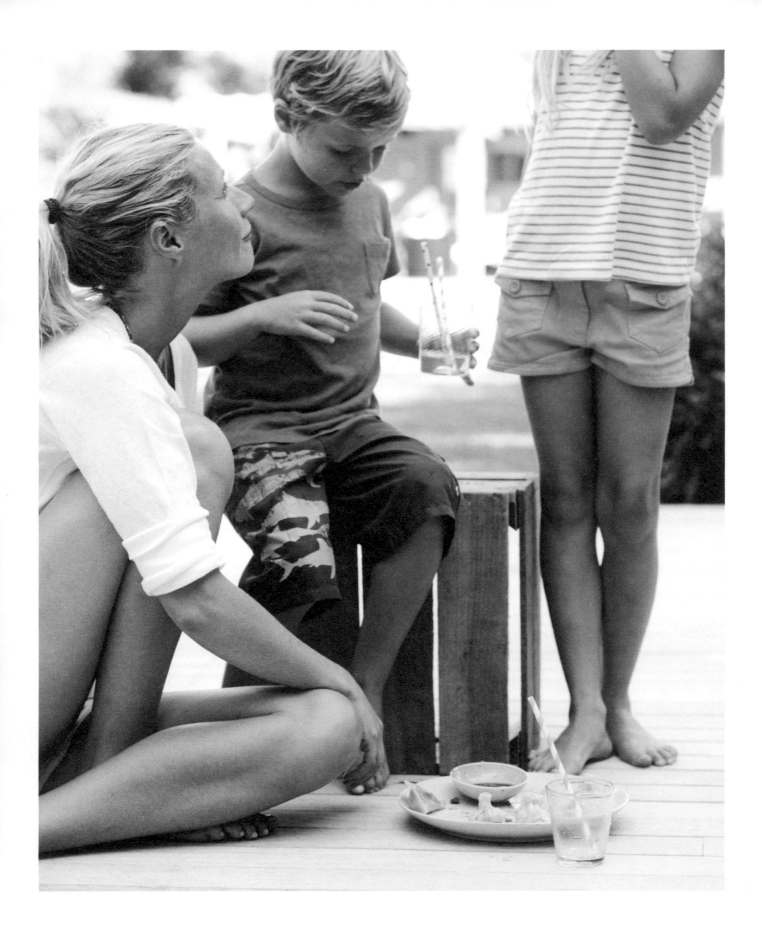

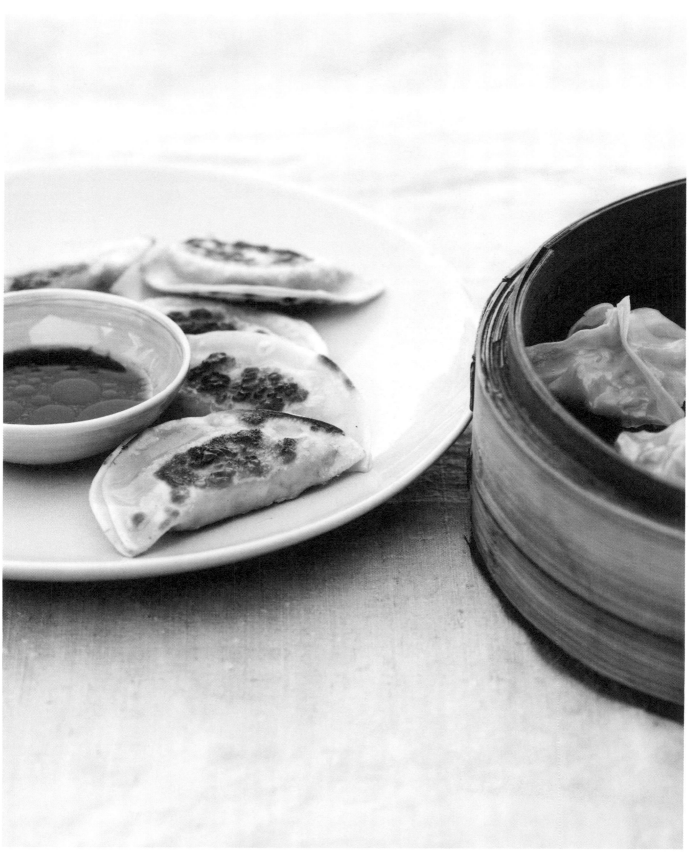

Veggie Dumplings (page 228), both pan-fried and steamed

FRESH VEGETABLES WITH PESTO MAYO

V Vegan

This doesn't even warrant a real recipe, but it's such a winner that we had to include it. Just mix a big spoonful of Vegenaise with a small spoonful of pesto (from a jar, or homemade, or maybe Classic Pesto on page 285—whatever) and serve alongside cut-up raw or steamed vegetables. Kids go nuts for pesto, and this is the easiest, fastest way I know to encourage them to get a few more veggies into their diet.

ROASTED CARROTS WITH HONEY + SOY SAUCE

The kids love these as much as I do. Come on, anything roasted with honey and soy is a winner.

Serves 4

V Vegan

8 carrots, peeled and cut into 2-inch lengths
2 tablespoons extra virgin olive oil
2 tablespoons manuka or raw honey
2 tablespoons soy sauce

Preheat your oven to 450°F and line a sheet pan with parchment paper.

Bring a large pot of salted water to a boil. Place the carrots in the water and cook until they just begin to lose their bite but aren't completely soft, 5 to 6 minutes. Meanwhile, whisk together the olive oil, honey, and soy sauce in a large mixing bowl. Drain the carrots thoroughly, add them to the bowl with the honey mixture, and stir to coat them evenly. Transfer the carrots to the prepared sheet pan and roast, stirring now and then, until completely caramelized, about 15 minutes. These are good served hot and at room temperature, too.

CHICKEN KABOBS

These super-easy chicken kabobs have good flavor and, because they come on a stick, appear very palatable to kids. Moses is a big fan.

Serves 4 kids

E Elimination Diet **P** Protein-Packed

¼ cup extra virgin olive oil
2 tablespoons freshly squeezed lemon juice
½ teaspoon coarse sea salt
1 large boneless, skinless organic chicken breast,
    cut into bite-sized cubes

Soak 4 wooden skewers in water for at least 10 minutes.

Meanwhile, whisk together the olive oil, lemon juice, and salt in a mixing bowl and add the chicken, stirring to coat. Let the chicken marinate, refrigerated, for at least 20 minutes and as long as overnight.

Heat a grill or grill pan over medium-high heat. Drain the skewers and evenly thread the chicken cubes onto them. Grill until firm to the touch and browned, about 3 minutes on each side. Serve immediately. These are really good with Pesto Mayo (see page 232), Lee's Hoisin Sauce (see page 275), or any of our salad dressings (see Salads + a Few Great Dressings, page 54).

BEST GLUTEN-FREE FISH FINGERS, TWO WAYS

Who doesn't love fish fingers? But as they're always dipped in a glutinous batter of some sort and deep fried, we had to think outside the box. Use packaged gluten-free bread crumbs or make your own. A good family dinner option is to serve these with a veggie of your choice and a delish salad.

Ⓟ Protein-Packed

MUSTARD + OLD BAY FISH FINGERS

¼ cup Vegenaise
2 tablespoons coarse seeded mustard
1 tablespoon Dijon mustard
1 cup plain gluten-free bread crumbs (purchased or made from well-toasted gluten-free bread blended in a powerful blender with salt, pepper, oregano, and some Old Bay Seasoning)
1 tablespoon Old Bay Seasoning
1 teaspoon fine sea salt
4 flounder, fluke, or sole fillets (or substitute skinless fillets of any flat, mild white fish), cut into 3-inch fingers
Olive oil spray
Lemon wedges for serving

Preheat the oven to 450°F and set on convection, if available. Line a baking sheet with parchment paper and set it aside.

Whisk together the Vegenaise and the mustards in a mixing bowl. In a separate bowl, whisk together the bread crumbs, Old Bay, and salt. Coat the fish fingers with the mustard mixture, then dredge them in the bread crumb mixture, tapping off any excess. Lay the fish fingers on the prepared baking sheet. Spray lightly with olive oil spray, turn fish fingers, and lightly spray the other side. Bake for 8 minutes, then turn the oven to broil and broil for 1 or 2 minutes, just to get the fish fingers nice and brown (if you don't have a broiler, just bake them for 10 minutes total). Serve immediately with plenty of lemon.

ITALIAN-STYLE FISH FINGERS

1 cup gluten-free plain bread crumbs (purchased or made from well-toasted gluten-free bread blended in a powerful blender with salt, pepper, oregano, and some Old Bay Seasoning)
1½ teaspoons dried oregano
1 teaspoon garlic powder
1 teaspoon fine sea salt
1 cup soy milk or rice milk
4 flounder, fluke, or sole fillets (or substitute skinless fillets of any flat, mild white fish), cut into fingers
Olive oil spray
Lemon wedges for serving

Preheat the oven to 450°F and set on convection, if available. Line a baking sheet with parchment paper and set it aside.

Whisk together the bread crumbs, oregano, garlic, and salt. Coat the fish fingers with the soy or rice milk, then dredge them in the bread crumb mixture, tapping off any excess. Lay the fish fingers on the prepared baking sheet. Spray lightly with olive oil spray, turn fish fingers, and lightly spray the other side. Bake for 8 minutes, then turn your oven to broil and broil for 1 or 2 minutes, just to get the fish fingers nice and brown (if you don't have a broiler, just bake them for 10 minutes total). Serve immediately with plenty of lemon.

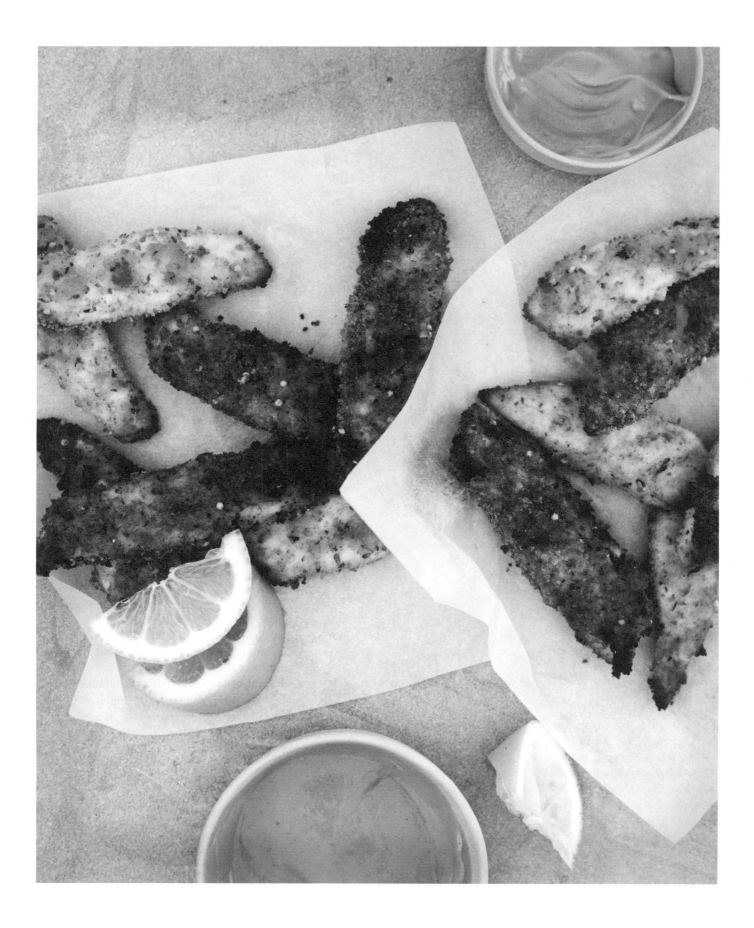

Some Notes on Crispy, Crunchy Nuggets

Julia and I do a lot of nuggets in our kitchens, and while we love the big crunch from the traditional triple dip through flour, egg, and bread crumbs (because, when all else fails, kids seem to eat whatever they're otherwise avoiding if it's crunchy), we usually employ a lighter hand.

Cut your protein—chicken, fish, even blocks of tofu—into bite-sized pieces.

For some glue, just do a quick swipe through a little almond, soy, or rice milk that you've added a big pinch of salt to. You can whisk in a bit of mustard for more flavor, or even some soy sauce or sesame oil.

Shake up your bread crumb routine. Try some of these alternatives: We like ground gluten-free pretzels (just whiz them in the food processor). Wasabi peas turn into a bright-green, super-crunchy crust. Or stick some gluten-free corn tortilla chips and pumpkin seeds in the food processor, or grind up your favorite gluten-free crackers. If you don't

feel like grinding anything, Mary's Gone Crackers sells gluten-free bread crumbs, which turn out really crunchy nuggets. You can also flavor your bread crumbs, as we do with the Old Bay in the fish fingers (see page 234).

Spritz your nuggets with olive oil and bake them, or shallow-fry them in a healthy oil (olive, canola, grapeseed, safflower). You can even use coconut oil for a little island-ish flavor.

We adore ketchup, don't get us wrong, but be creative with your nugget dips! Try maple syrup and mustard mixed together for pretzel-crusted chicken nuggets. Yum. Or Vegenaise thinned with soy sauce and a spoonful of miso for wasabi pea–crusted tofu nuggets…etc.

Think ahead! Any nugget can be breaded, lined up on a cookie sheet, frozen, and then stored in an airtight container in the freezer to be cooked anytime without defrosting. Dinner just got a lot easier!

CHICKEN FAJITAS

While trying to come up with ever more ways of cooking chicken within our guidelines, I had a eureka moment. These fajitas are totally yummy and flexible, and kids love them. If you're following an elimination regimen, skip the peppers, the chili powder, and the corn tortillas and serve with a side of black beans and brown rice. You won't realize you're on a diet.

Serves about 8 kids or a family of 4 generously

Ⓟ Protein-Packed

4 boneless, skinless chicken breasts, thinly sliced
Coarse sea salt
½ teaspoon freshly ground black pepper
1 tablespoon chili powder
1 teaspoon ground cumin
3 tablespoons extra virgin olive oil
1 red bell pepper, stem and seeds discarded,
    thinly sliced
1 orange bell pepper, stem and seeds discarded,
    thinly sliced
1 yellow onion, peeled and thinly sliced
Gluten-free tortillas for serving
Toppings: Guacamole (see page 243), Roasted
    Tomato + Chipotle Salsa (see page 282),
    hot sauce, lime wedges

In a large mixing bowl, thoroughly combine the chicken with a large pinch of salt, the black pepper, the chili powder, and the cumin. Set the chicken aside while you get your vegetables started.

Heat the olive oil over high heat in the largest nonstick skillet you've got. Add the peppers and onion and cook, stirring now and then, until they're beginning to soften, about 5 minutes. Add the seasoned chicken to the pan and cook on high, stirring now and then, until the chicken and vegetables are cooked through and nicely browned, 15 minutes.

Meanwhile, warm the tortillas. Serve them with the chicken and all the toppings and let everyone mix and match.

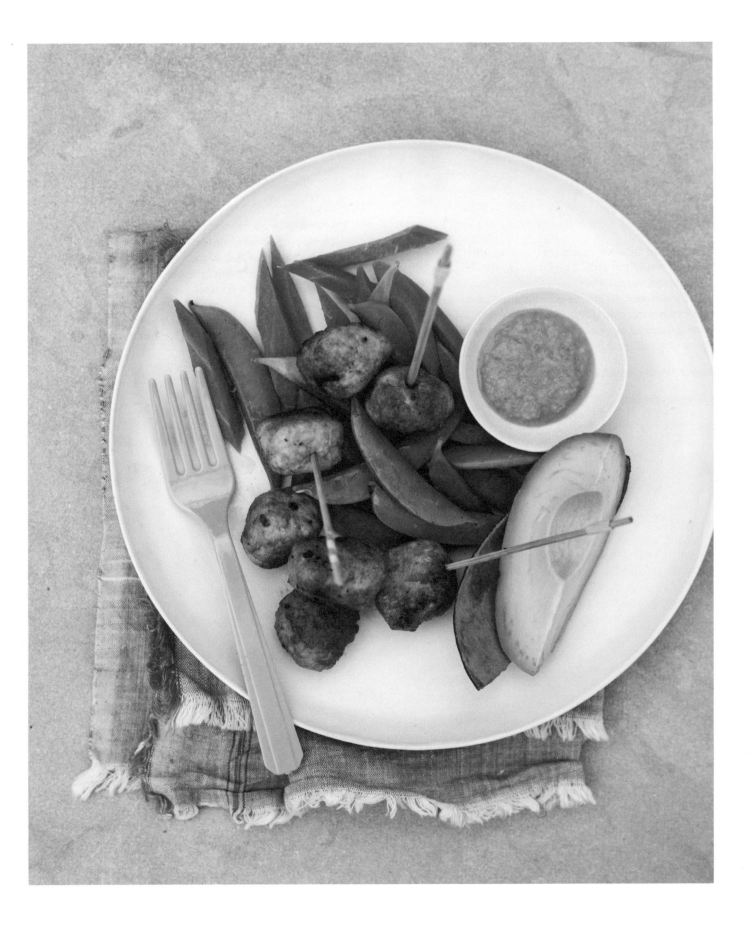

JAPANESE CHICKEN MEATBALLS

I have a hard time not gobbling these up when they're being served to the kids. They're so good! Very simple to prepare, and served with Lee's Hoisin Sauce (see page 275). Moses and his friends murder a big plate of these after kickboxing class. Turn these into a whole meal by serving them alongside cut-up vegetables to dip into Carrot-Ginger Dressing (see page 65).

Makes 2 dozen meatballs

P Protein-Packed

1 pound ground chicken (preferably dark meat)
½ teaspoon coarse sea salt
½ teaspoon freshly ground black pepper
1 garlic clove, very finely minced
1 teaspoon freshly grated ginger
1 tablespoon soy sauce
2 teaspoons good-quality maple syrup
2 tablespoons neutral oil (like canola, grapeseed, or safflower oil)
Lee's Hoisin Sauce (see page 275) for serving

Thoroughly mix the chicken with the salt, pepper, garlic, ginger, soy sauce, and maple syrup. Roll the mixture into golf ball–sized meatballs. Grill, roast, broil, or pan-fry the meatballs until they're cooked through and serve with Lee's Hoisin Sauce.

VEGAN SHEPHERD'S PIE

Made in a cupcake tin or little ramekins, these super-healthy, vegan, non-nightshade shepherd's pies go down like a treat. If your kids don't like the taste of parsnip, you can use mashed sweet potato or just regular ol' mashed white potatoes. If you use ramekins, be careful, because they get really hot—we wrap a napkin around each one so the kids don't burn their fingers.

Makes a dozen

V Vegan **P** Protein-Packed

FOR THE MASH (makes 4 cups)
Coarse sea salt
2 parsnips, peeled and roughly chopped (about
    2 cups)
1 small head of cauliflower, outer leaves and core
    discarded, roughly chopped (about 6 cups)
Coarse salt
½ cup soy milk
1 tablespoon extra virgin olive oil

FOR THE LENTILS (makes 2 cups)
¾ cup lentils (preferably the dark-green French
    variety called du Puy)
2 tablespoons extra virgin olive oil, plus a little
    extra for the ramekins
1 small red onion, peeled and finely diced (about
    1 cup)
1 carrot, peeled and finely diced
1 garlic clove, minced
1 teaspoon finely chopped fresh thyme
Coarse sea salt
5 tablespoons tomato paste
1½ tablespoons good-quality maple syrup

Bring a large pot of water to a boil and salt it generously. Add the parsnips and cauliflower and cook until they're very tender, 13 to 15 minutes. Drain the vegetables and return them to the pot, off the heat. Add a teaspoon of salt, the soy milk, and the olive oil and crush with a potato masher until very smooth.

Combine the lentils with 4 cups of water in a saucepan. Bring to a boil, lower the heat, and simmer until they're just soft, about 20 minutes. Drain and reserve the lentils.

Meanwhile, heat the olive oil in a small saucepan set over medium-high heat and add the onion, carrot, garlic, and thyme along with a healthy pinch of salt. Cook, stirring now and then, until softened but not browned, 10 minutes. Add the reserved lentils, another pinch of salt, the tomato paste, the maple syrup, and ½ cup water. Stir everything together and let it cook for an additional 5 minutes, just so all the flavors can meld. Season the mixture to taste with salt and set aside.

To bring it all together:

Preheat the oven to 350°F and set the rack in the upper third.

Line a 12-cup muffin tin with paper liners and evenly divide the lentils among the cups. Or divide among 12 lightly oiled ramekins. Top the lentils with the mash. Bake for 10 minutes (20 minutes if your lentils and mash are cold, ½ hour if they're frozen), then turn the oven to broil and cook just until the tops are browned. Serve immediately.

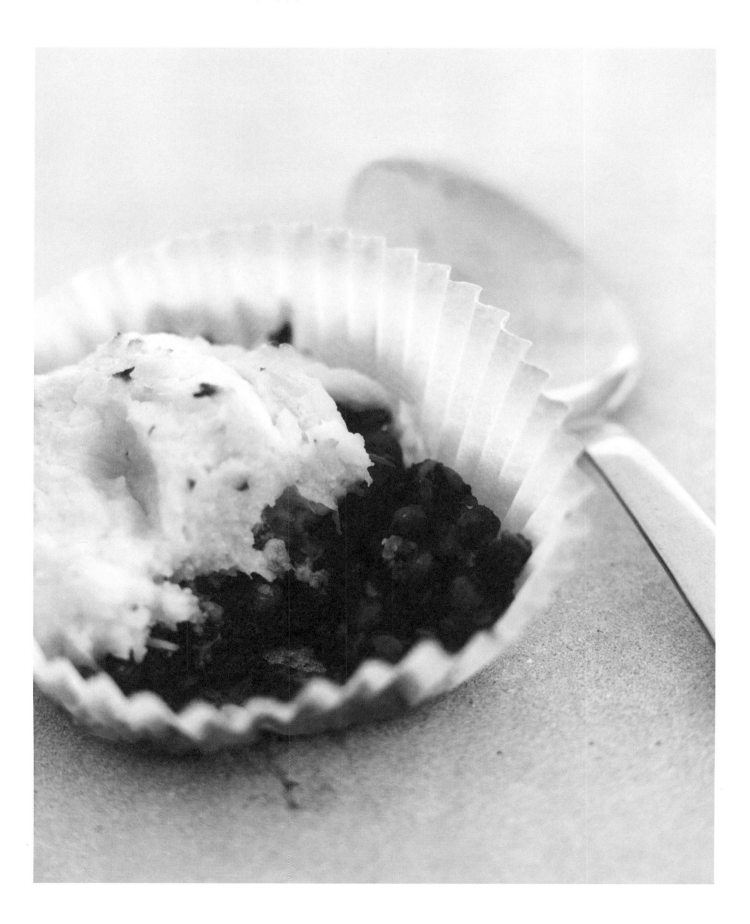

RICE CREAM SUNDAES

Based on the well-known Korean rice bowl called *bibimbap*, Rice Cream Sundaes are one of the best things we've created—the most rocking, flexible family meal ever.

Serves 4

V Vegan (depending on your toppings)
P Protein-Packed

Make a big batch of brown rice (or buckwheat soba noodles), then lay out lots of little bowls of whatever your kids like. I use diced avocado, steamed peas, broccoli sautéed with garlic and soy sauce, Savory Broiled Tofu (see recipe at right), shredded carrot—you get the idea. Kids have fun picking what they want to put on their grains from the "sundae" bar. For adults, we always include Salmon with Lee's Sriracha + Lime (see page 137) and fun veggies like Carrots with Black Sesame + Ginger (see page 161), Quick Cucumber Kimchi (see page 158), and Asian Greens with Garlic, Ginger + Fish Sauce (see page 162). Be sure to serve a bowl of Lee's Hoisin Sauce (see page 275) to drizzle over everything, and some thinly sliced scallions, too.

SAVORY BROILED TOFU

P Protein-Packed

Serves 4

¼ cup soy sauce
2 tablespoons raw honey
2 tablespoons extra virgin olive oil
2 teaspoons toasted sesame oil
2 small garlic cloves, finely minced
A 14-ounce box firm tofu, drained and cut into
　　½-inch cubes

Set your oven rack up close to your broiler and preheat the broiler to high.

Whisk together the soy sauce, honey, oils, and garlic in a mixing bowl. Add the tofu to the bowl and gently stir to coat it with the mixture. Transfer the tofu to a baking sheet and pour over it whatever liquid remains in the bowl. Broil, stirring now and then, until the tofu is browned and has a few crispy edges, just 4 to 5 minutes total, depending on the heat of your broiler.

BLACK BEAN + GUACAMOLE TACOS

These are super-easy and make my kids really happy. Keep fresh corn tortillas in the freezer, placing a piece of parchment paper between them and wrapping them in plastic or putting them in a zip-top bag—that way you can defrost just as many as you need. Apple and Moses like to add hot sauce to their tacos.

Serves 4 kids (makes 8 tacos)

Ⓥ Vegan Ⓟ Protein-Packed

Go-To Black Beans (see page 275)
2 ripe avocados
2 tablespoons minced white onion
3 tablespoons roughly chopped cilantro
1 lime
Coarse sea salt
8 corn tortillas

Warm the beans over low heat.

Cut each avocado in half, remove and discard the pits, and score the flesh inside the shells. Scoop the avocado into a mixing bowl and mash gently with a fork—you don't want it to be completely smooth. Stir in the onion and cilantro. Cut the lime in half and squeeze in juice to taste. Season the guacamole to taste with salt.

Warm a corn tortilla in a dry skillet and serve with a generous swipe of guacamole and a spoonful of beans. Repeat over and over again, because kids *love these*.

CAMERINO'S POPCORN

Our dear friend Cameron is a master popcorn maker—and this is one of the many reasons she is Apple and Mosey's favorite houseguest. We use organic kernels and follow her directions for the best hot popcorn ever—perfect for a movie night.

Makes about 15 cups

Ⓥ Vegan

Extra virgin olive oil
½ cup organic popcorn kernels
Coarse sea salt

Set a large, heavy pot over high heat. Add enough olive oil to generously coat the bottom of the pot and let the oil get very, very hot, nearly smoking. Add the popcorn kernels and cover the pot with a tight-fitting lid. Shake the pot to coat the kernels with oil and let the heat do its thing. When the aggressive popping sound just begins to subside, remove the pot from the heat and carefully take off the lid. Transfer the popcorn to a large mixing bowl and season to taste with plenty of salt. Serve immediately, preferably with a very fun film.

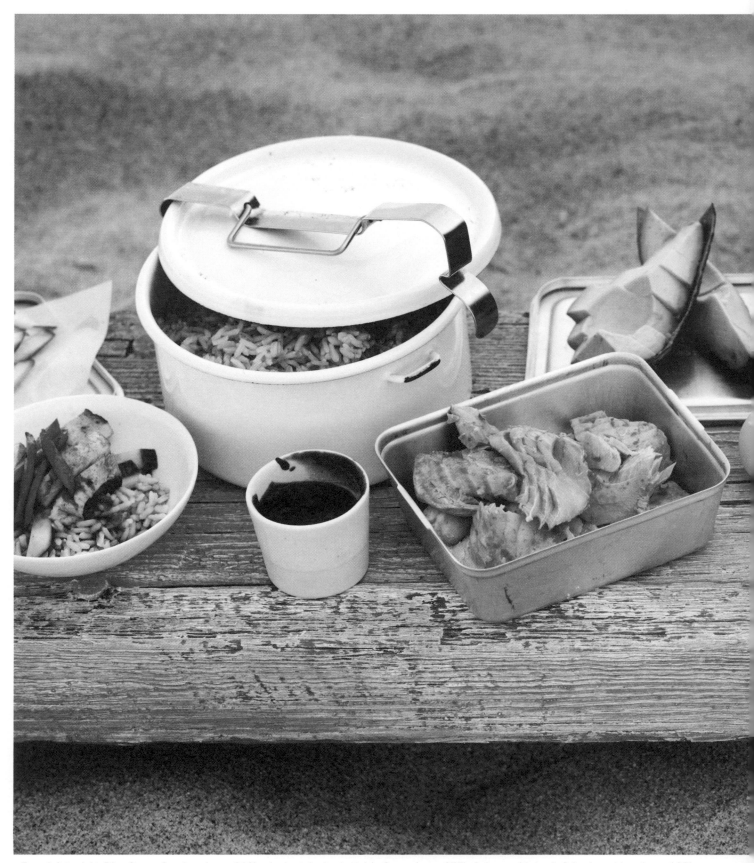

From left to right, Rice Cream Sundaes (page 242), picnic style; Lee's Hoisin Sauce (page 275); Salmon with Lee's Sriracha + Lime (page 137); avocado; Carrots with Black Sesame + Ginger (page 161); tomatoes; snap peas; Savory Broiled Tofu (page 242)

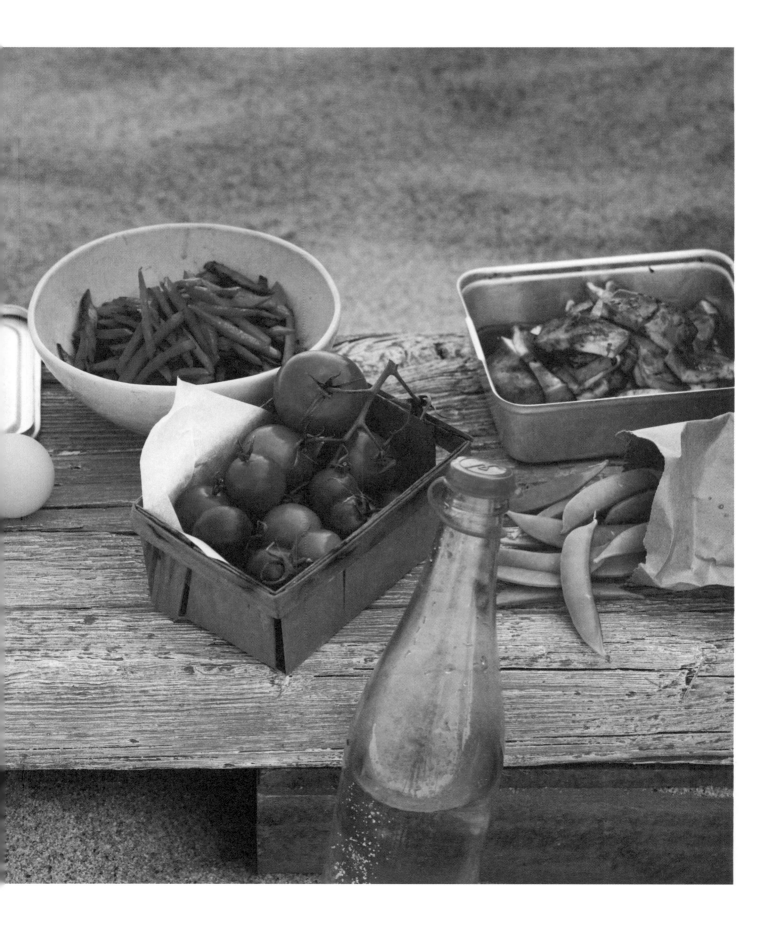

KALE CHIPS

These kale chips are in *My Father's Daughter,* but I also had to include them here. Kale—or any dark leafy green, for that matter—can be tough to get kids to eat, but when these chips hit the table, the kids forget it's kale. These can also be jazzed up with lemon or lime juice, crushed red chili flakes, pimentón, curry powder, even hippie-dippie nutritional yeast, which makes them kinda like Doritos…kinda. If you use any of these flavors, it's best to mix by hand after the kale leaves are coated in oil so that the seasoning gets evenly distributed.

Serves 4

Ⓔ Elimination Diet **Ⓥ** Vegan

**1 big bunch of kale, stems discarded and
     leaves torn into roughly 1½-inch pieces
2 tablespoons extra virgin olive oil
Coarse sea salt**

Preheat the oven to 400°F. Toss the kale with the olive oil and spread out on 2 baking sheets. Sprinkle with coarse salt and roast, stirring occasionally, for 12 to 15 minutes, or until light brown and crispy. Eat like potato chips.

AMAGANSETT APPLESAUCE

We have apple trees at our house in Amagansett, New York, and in October they're bursting with fruit. I search for ways to use the apples up, making apple juice, baked apples, apple crumble, and, of course, applesauce for the kids. I use tart-ish apples to make this perfect fall after-school snack or dessert.

Makes 2 to 3 cups

Ⓔ Elimination Diet **Ⓥ** Vegan

**4 kinda sweet, kinda tart apples (we like
     Honeycrisps)**

Peel and core the apples and discard the trimmings. Roughly chop the apples and put them in a small saucepan with a splash of water. Bring the mixture to a boil, turn the heat to low, and simmer until the apples give off plenty of their own juice and are really soft, about 15 minutes (depending on the type of apple). Crush with a potato masher and serve warm or at room temperature.

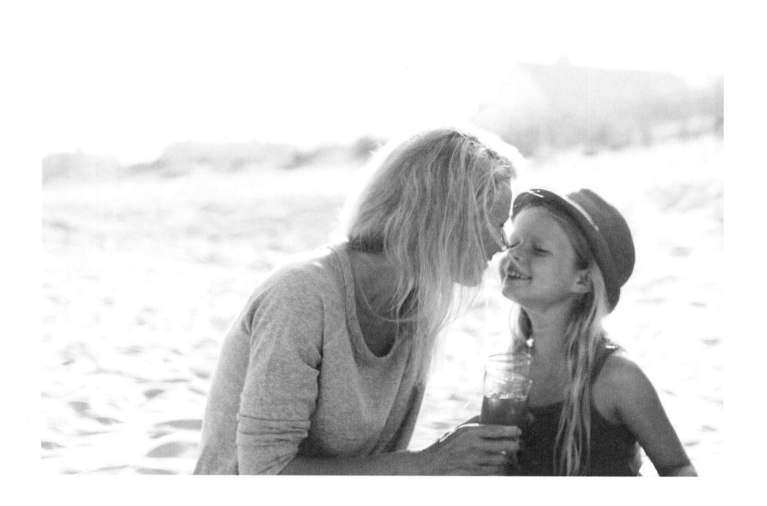

SWEET TOOTH

For this chapter we set our minds and taste buds to coming up with sweets that will not be bad for you—the most challenging aspect of any healthy eating plan. We all know that sugar is unhealthy and that it's good to steer clear of dairy and wheat. But then, how do you make a cake? Or ice cream? What do you eat when you're craving something sweet and the rules keep changing (last year agave was the miracle sweetener, now it's not so good)? We've worked to compile recipes that will satisfy any sweet tooth while keeping them on the straight and narrow. And we've had a lot of help from our favorite pastry chef, Darleen Gross, who redefines how good healthy treats can be.

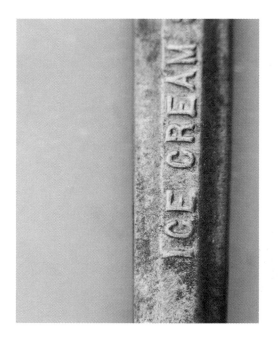

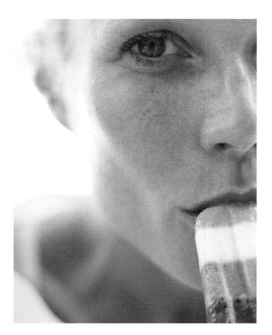

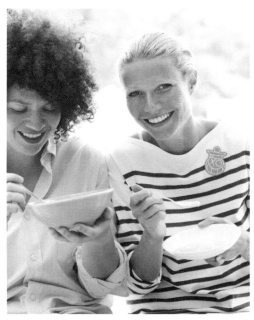

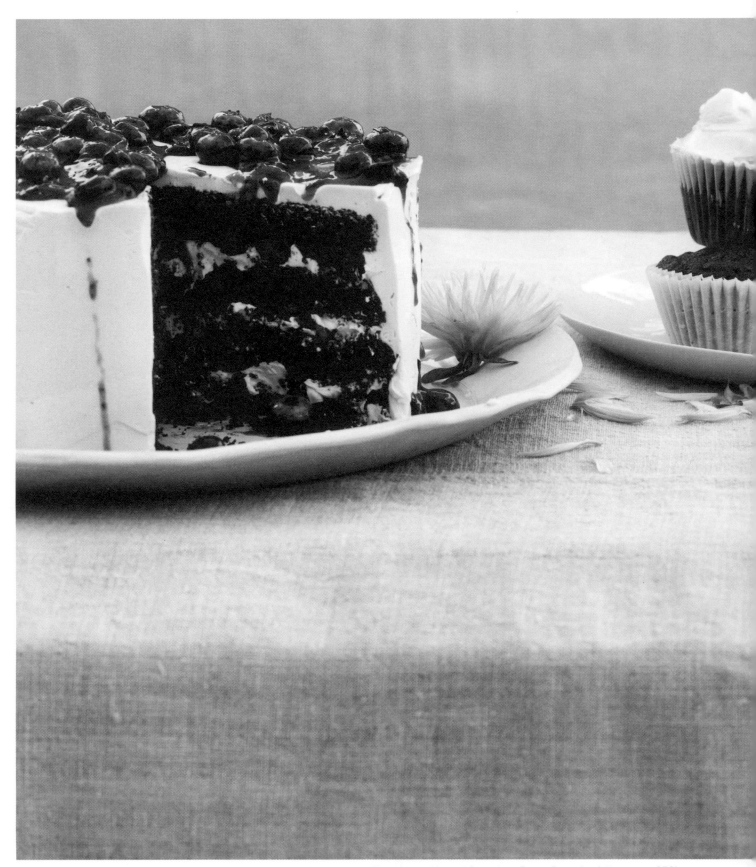

From left to right: Chocolate Cake with Darleen's Healthy Buttercream; Chocolate + Almond Cupcakes; Power Brownies (all on page 253)

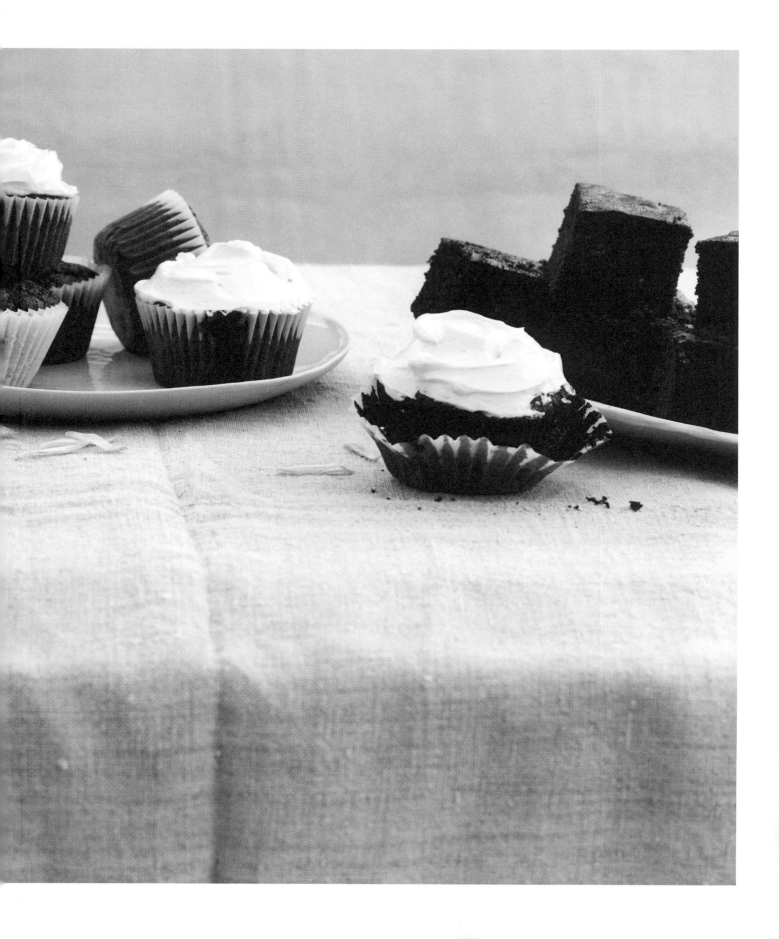

DARK CHOCOLATE BARK WITH COCONUT, ALMONDS + SEA SALT

Dark chocolate is super-rich in antioxidants; it's a real superfood. Here we turn it into an extremely appealing bark that you can flavor in a variety of ways—feel free to mix up the toppings and use whatever nuts, dried fruit, and spices you like (dried cherries and spicy red chili flakes, hazelnuts combined with sliced dried apricots…). This is perfect as a snack when you want a little something sweet, or cracked into pieces and served at the end of a meal.

Serves 4 as a snack

Ⓥ Vegan

7 ounces good-quality dark chocolate (we like
    Green + Black's 70% bars), roughly chopped
2 tablespoons sliced almonds
2 tablespoons unsweetened coconut flakes
1 teaspoon Maldon sea salt

Line a sheet pan with a piece of parchment paper and set it aside.

Bring a small pot of water to a boil, then lower the heat to a simmer. Put the chocolate in a glass or stainless steel bowl and set it over the pot of water. Stir the chocolate until it's completely melted and immediately pour it onto the prepared pan. Evenly sprinkle the almonds, coconut, and salt over the chocolate. Put the pan in the freezer until the chocolate sets, about 15 minutes. Break the chocolate into pieces and eat immediately, or store at room temperature in an airtight container if your house is cool, or in the refrigerator if it's summertime!

THE BROWNIE RECIPE THAT COULD

I swear by this cakey brownie recipe, originally in *My Father's Daughter*. Here we use the tried-and-tested batter and jazz it up in a few new ways. See the variations below.

Ⓥ Vegan

BASIC BROWNIE RECIPE

Makes 12 to18 brownies, depending on how big you cut them

2 cups white spelt flour, if you can tolerate a little
    gluten, or all-purpose gluten-free flour
    (if the flour doesn't include xanthan gum,
    add 1 teaspoon)
1 cup high-quality cocoa powder
1½ tablespoons baking powder
A pinch of fine sea salt
½ cup Vegenaise or vegetable oil
1 cup good-quality maple syrup
½ cup brown rice syrup
½ cup strong brewed coffee
½ cup soy milk or rice milk
1 tablespoon pure vanilla extract

Preheat the oven to 350°F. Line a baking dish (we use a 9 x 11-inch dish that's 2 inches high) with parchment paper and lightly oil the parchment with a neutral oil.

Sift the flour, cocoa, baking powder, and salt together in a large mixing bowl. In a separate bowl, whisk together the Vegenaise or oil, the syrups, the coffee, the soy milk, and the vanilla. Mix the wet ingredients into the dry ones, being careful not to overbeat (that's how you end up with a tough brownie!). Pour the batter into the prepared baking dish. Bake for 30 minutes (less if your pan is shallow, more if it's deep), or until a toothpick comes out with just a bit of chocolate on it (this means the brownies will be super-fudgy). Let the brownies cool before cutting into squares. Serve right away, or store in an airtight container.

VARIATIONS USING THE BASIC BROWNIE RECIPE

POWER BROWNIES

Ⓟ Protein-Packed

Add 4 servings of plain whey protein powder to the Basic Brownie Recipe batter along with ⅓ cup ground flaxseeds and bake as directed above.

CHOCOLATE + ALMOND CUPCAKES

Ⓥ Vegan Ⓟ Protein-Packed

For Reese's-esque cupcakes: Prepare the Basic Brownie Recipe batter. Combine ¼ cup roasted almond butter and ¼ cup good-quality maple syrup and set the mixture aside. Line a standard 12-cup muffin tin with paper liners. Fill each muffin cup halfway with the brownie batter. Evenly divide the almond butter–maple syrup mixture among the muffin cups and top with the remaining batter. Bake at 350°F for 25 minutes. Let cool completely before serving.

CHOCOLATE CAKE WITH DARLEEN'S HEALTHY BUTTERCREAM

Ⓥ Vegan

Prepare the Basic Brownie Recipe batter and divide it between two greased 8- or 9-inch cake tins. Bake at 350°F for 20 minutes. Let the cakes cool completely before frosting with Darleen's Healthy Buttercream (at right). We like to do this as a double-layer cake with frosting between the layers and then all around and on top of the tall cake. Feel free to add fresh berries between the layers and on top, too!

DARLEEN'S HEALTHY BUTTERCREAM

Makes 4 cups

Ⓥ Vegan

2 cups Spectrum organic shortening (nonhydrogenated palm oil, available at Whole Foods)
1 cup tapioca starch
1 cup agave nectar (or grade A light maple syrup)
1 tablespoon pure vanilla extract (the vanilla contributes to the slightly beige color; if you want a brighter white, you can substitute vanilla-flavored Stevia drops—just a few drops, as they'll add sweetness!)

Place all the ingredients in the bowl of an electric mixer and beat with the whisk attachment until light and fluffy. The frosting can be refrigerated for up to a month, but bring it back to room temperature and rewhip it before using.

BUMMER BARS

My best friend, Mary, sometimes sets up a secret, roving bakery in East Los Angeles called Treat Street. It's a flour, sugar, and icing extravaganza, and it's the best. But as it's in Los Angeles, she has to include something vegan, something sugar/dairy/gluten free. One day her friend Andy lovingly called this class of treat Bummer Bars, and the name stuck. I love a good Bummer Bar.

Ⓥ Vegan Ⓟ Protein-Packed

1½ cups quinoa flakes
¼ cup ground flaxseeds
A pinch of fine sea salt
¼ teaspoon ground cinnamon
¼ teaspoon ground nutmeg
½ teaspoon ground ginger
¼ cup extra virgin olive oil
¼ cup good-quality maple syrup
2 tablespoons brown rice syrup
½ cup chopped prunes or apricots
½ cup chopped pecans or walnuts

Preheat the oven to 350°F. Line a brownie pan (we use a 9 x 11-inch dish that's 2 inches high) with parchment paper or line a 12-cup muffin tin with paper liners.

Combine all the ingredients in a large bowl and pour the mixture into the brownie pan, or evenly divide it among the muffin cups. Pack the mixture down with a rubber spatula. Bake for ½ hour, or until the bars have firmed up and are golden brown. Let cool before removing from the pan or muffin cups. If you used a brownie pan, use the parchment to lift the bar out of the pan, and cut into rectangles. Serve right away or store in an airtight container.

CANDY BARS!

Darleen devised these decadent candy bars, and all the chocoholics in my house flipped for them—we can't get enough. The bars keep well in the refrigerator for up to 2 weeks, and we even like them frozen!

Makes about 1½ dozen bars

Ⓥ Vegan

1½ cups raw cashews
1½ cups dates, pitted and roughly chopped
½ cup almond butter
½ cup grade B maple syrup
½ cup coconut flour
½ cup unsweetened shredded coconut
½ teaspoon almond extract
1½ cups dark chocolate chips (60% or higher
    cocoa content)
1½ tablespoons coconut oil

Grind the cashews to a very fine meal in a food processor. Add the dates, almond butter, maple syrup, coconut flour, shredded coconut, and almond extract and pulse until you have a sticky ball of dough.

Line a small sheet pan with parchment paper and press the cashew mixture out onto the paper, making a rectangle 1 inch deep. It helps if you put a drop of oil or water on your hands before doing this. Refrigerate the mixture for 6 to 8 hours, until it's firm.

Meanwhile, combine the chocolate chips and coconut oil in a stainless steel or glass bowl set over a pot of simmering water (make sure the water doesn't touch the bowl). Stir the mixture until it's just melted, remove the bowl from the heat, and pour the chocolate mixture over the cold cashew mixture. Return the bar to the fridge and let it cool until the chocolate coating is set, at least 1 hour.

Using the parchment, lift the bar out of the sheet pan and cut it into rectangles (or you can use cookie cutters to make fun shapes for kids!). Serve at once, or store in an airtight container.

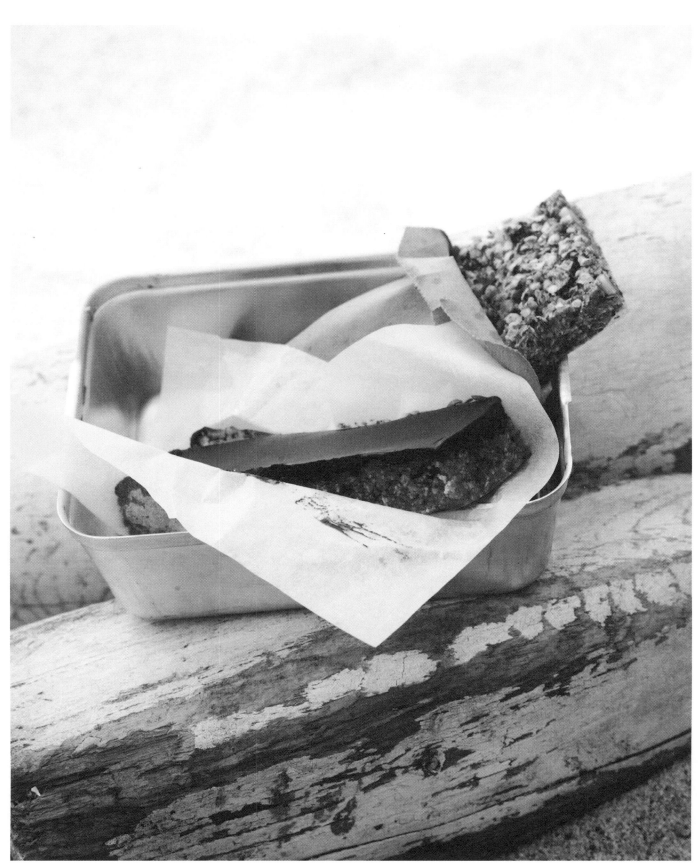

Candy Bar (in front),-Bummer Bar (in back)

SUMMER FRUIT PARFAIT

A colorful, delicious dessert, this is Darleen's vegan masterpiece. It's quite a bit of work to make these parfaits, but it's really fun to get creative with such interesting ingredients, and the results are just stunning.

Serves 6

Ⓥ Vegan

FOR THE STRAWBERRY JELL
2 cups apple juice
2 tablespoons agar flakes (available at Whole Foods, health food stores, and online)
A pinch of sea salt
2 teaspoons kuzu root starch or 1 tablespoon arrowroot (available at Whole Foods, health food stores, and online)
1 tablespoon water
2 cups fresh strawberries, stems discarded

FOR THE APRICOT JELL
2½ cups apricot nectar
2 tablespoons agar flakes
A pinch of sea salt
2 teaspoons kuzu root starch or 1 tablespoon arrowroot
2 tablespoons water

FOR THE ALMOND WHIP
1¼ cups almond meal or 1 cup raw blanched almonds finely ground in a food processor
1 cup boiling water
2 tablespoons grade B maple syrup
2 cups cool water, plus 2 tablespoons (divided)
Seeds from ½ vanilla bean
3 tablespoons agar flakes
A pinch of sea salt
1 tablespoon kuzu root starch or 1½ tablespoons arrowroot
½ cup grade A light maple syrup or agave nectar

FOR THE PARFAITS
2 pints assorted fresh berries
3 or 4 fresh apricots, peaches, or nectarines

To make the Strawberry Jell: Pour the apple juice into a saucepan and sprinkle the agar flakes over the top. Let the mixture stand for 10 minutes to allow the agar to soften. Bring the mixture to a boil over medium heat and add the salt. Turn the heat to low and simmer, stirring, until the agar is dissolved, 10 to 15 minutes.

Whisk the kuzu root or arrowroot with the water in a small bowl to make a slurry, then quickly stir the slurry into the juice. If you're using kuzu, return the mixture to a boil and cook for 3 minutes; if you're using arrowroot, remove it from the heat once it reaches the boil. Combine the apple juice mixture with the berries in a large mixing bowl and chill in the refrigerator for 1 to 2 hours. Once the mixture is firm, scoop it into a blender and puree until smooth, scraping down the sides as needed. Chill until ready to serve.

To make the Apricot Jell: Place the apricot nectar in a small saucepan and sprinkle the agar flakes over the top. Let the mixture stand for 10 minutes to allow the agar to soften. Bring the mixture to a boil over medium heat and add the salt. Turn the heat to low and simmer, stirring, until the agar is dissolved, 10 to 15 minutes.

Whisk the kuzu root or arrowroot with the water in a small bowl to make a slurry, then quickly stir the slurry into the juice. If you're using kuzu, return the mixture to a boil and cook for 3 minutes; if you're using arrowroot, remove it from the heat once it reaches the boil. Pour the mixture into a shallow bowl and chill in the refrigerator for 1 to 2 hours. Once the mixture is firm, scoop it into a blender and puree until smooth, scraping down the sides as needed. Chill until ready to serve.

To make the Almond Whip: Place the almond meal or ground almonds, boiling water, and grade B maple syrup in a powerful blender and blend until they form a smooth paste. Add the 2 cups water, blending on high, until creamy. Pour the almond milk through a fine-mesh strainer into a clean saucepan and discard the pulp.

Add the vanilla and salt to the almond milk and sprinkle the agar flakes over the mixture. Let the mixture stand for 10 minutes to allow the agar to soften. Bring the mixture to a boil over medium heat and add the salt. Turn the heat to low and simmer, stirring, until the agar is dissolved, 10 to 15 minutes.

Whisk the kuzu root or arrowroot with the 2 reserved tablespoons of water in a small bowl to make a slurry, then quickly stir the slurry into the almond milk. If you're using kuzu, return the mixture to a boil and cook for 3 minutes; if you're using arrowroot, remove it from the heat once it reaches the boil. Whisk in the light maple syrup or agave. Pour the mixture through a fine-mesh strainer into a glass bowl or casserole dish and refrigerate uncovered until set (it will be quite firm), about 2 hours. Once it's set, scoop the almond mixture into the blender and blend on medium speed until completely smooth, stopping to scrape down the sides as needed. When it's smooth, spoon it into an airtight container and refrigerate until ready to use.

To assemble the parfaits: Alternate layers of the fresh fruit with the Almond Whip, the Strawberry Jell, and the Apricot Jell, dividing all evenly among 6 parfait glasses. Finish each with a dollop of Almond Whip. If you like a bit of crunchy texture, sprinkle in a layer or 2 of your favorite granola, cookie crumbs, or chopped roasted nuts. Keep chilled until ready to serve.

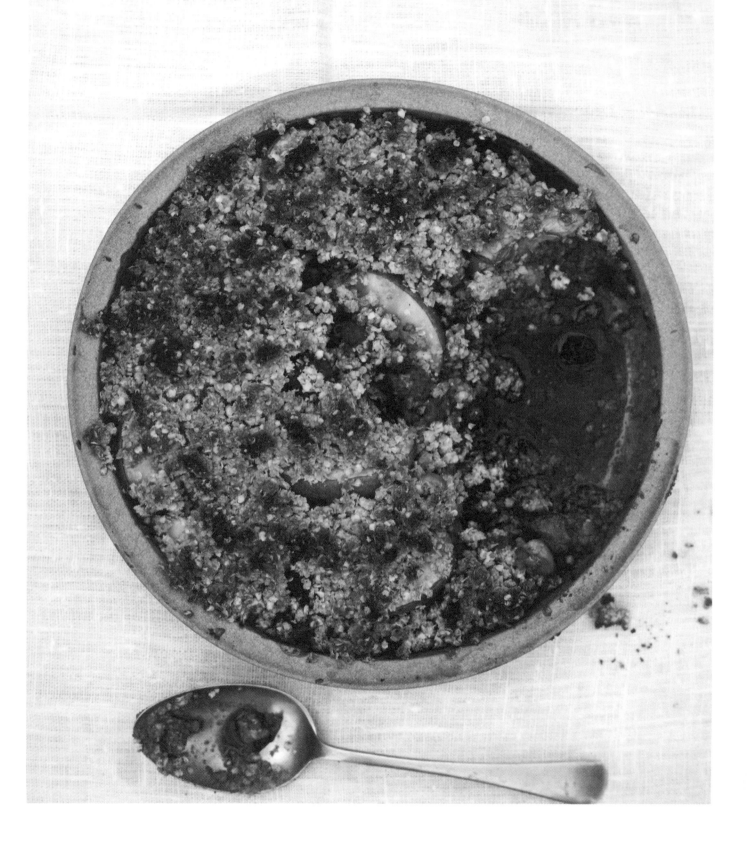

FLOURLESS ANYTHING CRUMBLE

Crumble is always a nostalgic crowd-pleaser. You don't even have to mention the flourless/sugarless part with this one—no one can ever tell. This recipe is great with stone fruit and berries (try mixing white raspberries with fresh apricots, or sliced nectarines with blueberries).

Serves 6

Ⓥ Vegan Ⓟ Protein-Packed

4 cups fruit (peeled and sliced stone fruit, berries, whatever)
4 tablespoons good-quality maple syrup, divided
1 tablespoon freshly squeezed lemon juice
½ cup almond meal (or grind ½ cup of blanched almonds in a powerful blender until they're powdery)
½ cup quinoa flakes
A pinch of fine sea salt
½ teaspoon ground cinnamon (or any dessert spice—try cardamom and clove with chopped pears, for example)
2 tablespoons extra virgin olive oil

Preheat the oven to 400°F.

Toss the fruit in a shallow baking dish with 2 tablespoons of the maple syrup and the lemon juice. Mix the almond meal, quinoa flakes, salt, and cinnamon in a large bowl. Add the 2 remaining tablespoons of maple syrup and the olive oil and mix until just combined. Crumble the mixture over the fruit and bake until the topping is browned and the fruit is bubbling, 20 to 25 minutes.

NORI SESAME CRUNCH

A salty-sweet snack, this treat is easy to prepare and is lovely alongside a cup of green tea or a spicy chai.

Makes 12

Ⓥ Vegan

3 sheets untoasted nori seaweed
½ cup Just-Like-Honey syrup (a rice-based sweetener made and distributed by Suzanne's Specialties)
½ cup white and/or black sesame seeds

Preheat the oven to 350°F and line a sheet pan with a piece of parchment paper.

Use scissors to cut each nori sheet into 4 long strips; make sure your hands are dry or the nori will soften. Pour the syrup into a wide, shallow bowl and pour the seeds onto a large plate. Take a nori strip and, with the textured side down, drag it across the surface of the syrup, leaving ½ inch dry for gripping. Scrape off the excess syrup with the straight edge of a metal spatula so there's just the thinnest coating; if it's too heavy, the strips will curl in the oven. Press evenly into the seeds and place, seed side up, on the prepared pan.

Bake the strips for 10 minutes, then lift them off the pan and transfer them to a wire rack to cool and crisp. Once they've cooled, if you find they're chewy, return them to the oven on the wire rack and bake for 3 to 5 minutes more. Let cool. Store in an airtight container for up to 2 weeks.

ALMOND BUTTER COOKIES WITH MALDON SALT

Often when I'm doing an elimination diet, what I miss most is the crunch of biting into something made with flour and then baked. These amazing treats bring you all the satisfaction of cookies, with no guilt! The Maldon salt really takes them to the next level by giving you that sea-salt-and-caramel sweet-and-savory combo. I once overnighted a batch from London to my manager in Los Angeles who was doing the clean program and was dying for a cookie! They did not disappoint. These cookies can be eaten any time of day.

Makes about 2 dozen

V Vegan **P** Protein-Packed

1½ cups gluten-free flour (if the flour doesn't
    include xanthan gum, add ¾ teaspoon)
½ teaspoon fine sea salt
1 teaspoon baking powder
1 cup natural almond butter
1 cup good-quality maple syrup
1 teaspoon pure vanilla extract
½ teaspoon Maldon sea salt (or you can use
    fleur de sel or any coarse sea salt you
    have on hand)

Preheat the oven to 350°F and line 2 baking sheets with parchment paper.

Whisk together the flour, fine sea salt, and baking powder. In a separate bowl, whisk together the almond butter, maple syrup, and vanilla. Thoroughly combine the wet and dry ingredients. Using 2 spoons, form the cookies into small balls (each about 1 generous tablespoon) and space them 2 inches apart on the prepared sheet pans. Wet your fingertips and press down on each cookie, smoothing the edges so each is a nice little disk. Sprinkle each cookie with just a bit of the Maldon salt.

Bake until the air is fragrant and the cookies are just firm, 10 to 12 minutes. Let them cool on a rack before serving.

BANANA "ICE CREAM" WITH SWEET-AND-SALTY ROASTED ALMONDS

This recipe has all the rich, creamy texture of ice cream with none of the dairy or sugar. The crunchy topping is a snap to put together and is so, so good.

Makes about 1 pint

Ⓥ Vegan

4 ripe bananas, peeled and sliced into thin
    rounds
¼ cup finely chopped roasted almonds
2 teaspoons plus 2 tablespoons good-quality
    maple syrup, divided
A pinch of coarse sea salt
½ cup unsweetened almond milk
1 teaspoon pure vanilla extract

Freeze the banana slices in a single layer on a tray or plate lined with parchment or wax paper. Once the slices are frozen, use them immediately or keep frozen in a zip-top plastic bag or airtight container for up to a month.

Meanwhile, in a small bowl, combine the almonds with 2 teaspoons of the maple syrup and the pinch of salt and set the mixture aside.

Combine the frozen banana slices, the almond milk, the remaining 2 tablespoons of the maple syrup, and the vanilla in a food processor and pulse until the mixture is the texture of soft-serve ice cream, scraping down the sides as necessary. Don't worry if the mixture is not totally smooth at first—once the bananas start to break down and defrost in the food processor, they'll give in and the "ice cream" will take shape quickly.

Spoon the banana "ice cream" into bowls immediately and sprinkle each serving with a bit of the almond mixture.

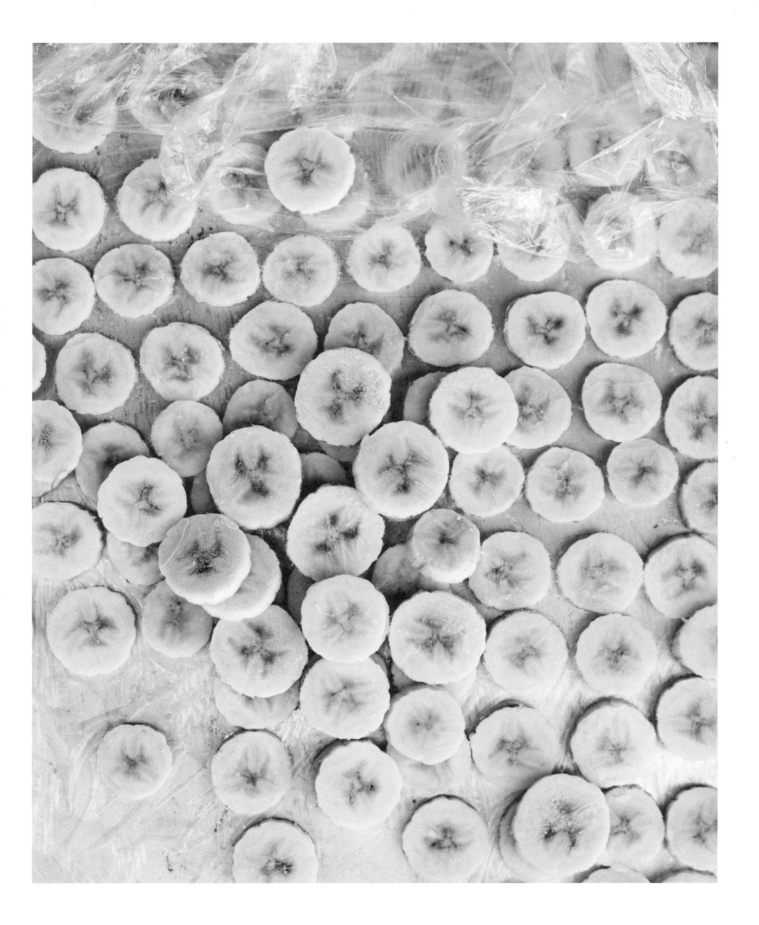

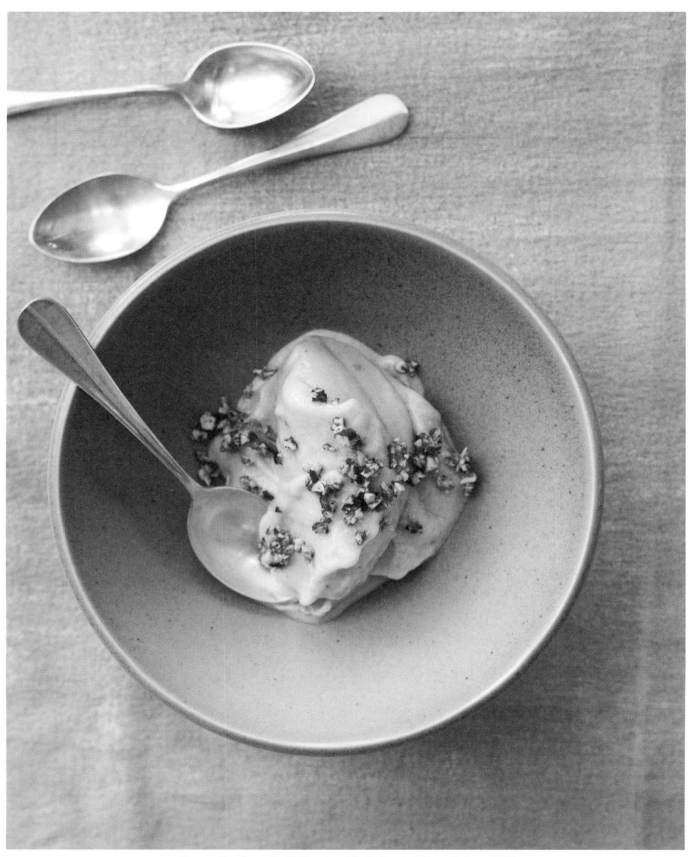

Banana "Ice Cream" with Sweet-and-Salty Roasted Almonds (page 261)

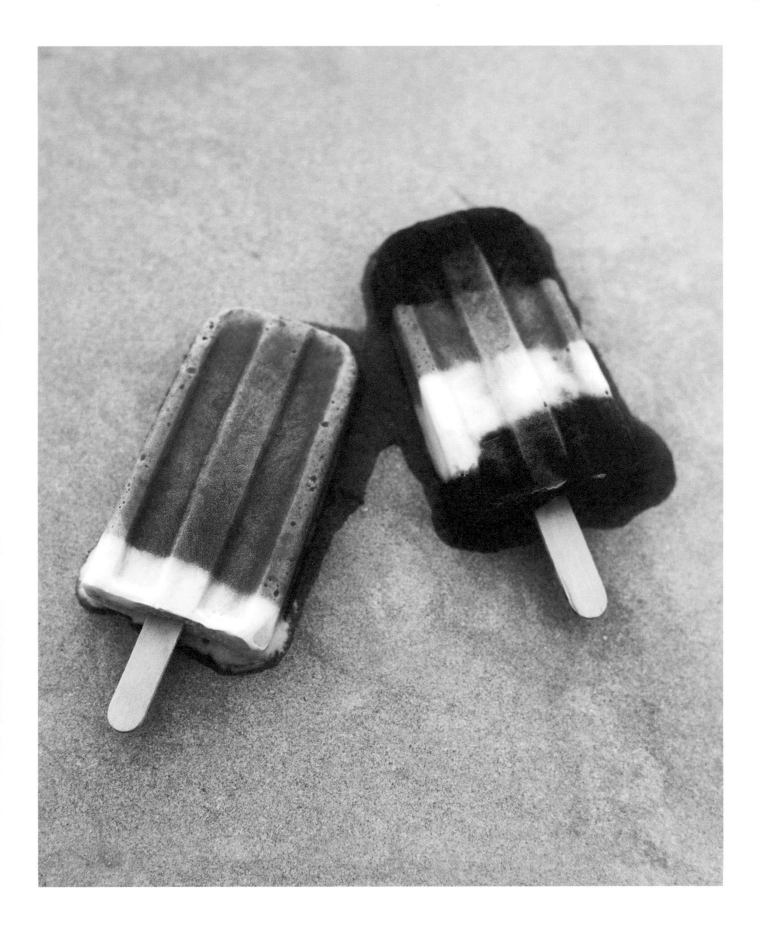

INSTANT BERRY + COCONUT SHERBET (OR FROZEN POPS!)

So easy, so fresh, so sweet, vegan, and sugar-free, this is the perfect dessert to make when you've forgotten to make dessert.

Makes 1 pint

V Vegan

2 cups frozen berries (whatever type you like; we
    like a mix of blueberries, blackberries, and
    raspberries)
½ cup coconut milk
2 tablespoons good-quality maple syrup

Combine everything in a food processor and pulse until completely smooth. Eat immediately—at this point it's got the perfect soft texture. Or freeze and then let it sit at room temperature for about 10 minutes to soften a bit before serving.

FOR FROZEN POPS

Use the same ratios as above, but substitute fresh berries for frozen ones and pour the puree into frozen-pop molds. If you've got time, make batches of individual berry flavors (strawberry, blackberry, raspberry, etc.) and freeze them in stripes, using a bit of plain coconut milk between the layers if you like. Kids go crazy for these!

FAVORITE BAKED APPLES

My favorite singer grew up in the English countryside where the apples are tart and abundant. His mom used to make baked apples, and here is my version. Perfect in autumn.

Serves 6

E Elimination Diet (leave out the raisins and maple syrup)
V Vegan

½ cup raisins
½ cup chopped walnuts
1 teaspoon ground cinnamon
A pinch of fine sea salt
3 tablespoons good-quality maple syrup
6 apples (we especially like Honeycrisps
     for this, but whichever are
     your favorite), cored

Preheat the oven to 350°F.

Mix together the raisins, walnuts, cinnamon, salt, and maple syrup in a small bowl. Place the apples in a baking dish and stuff each with an equal amount of the raisin and walnut mixture. Bake until the apples are soft, 35 to 45 minutes, depending on what variety of apple you're using. Serve hot, warm, or at room temperature, being sure to spoon the juice from the baking dish over the apples.

DARLEEN'S DARK CHOCOLATE PUDDING

This simple, intense, wonderfully chocolaty chocolate pudding is, remarkably, completely vegan. A genius when it comes to making familiar, comforting desserts better for us, Darleen swaps rich dairy for a quick whirl in the blender or food processor to make this pudding beautifully creamy. Try it adorned with a spoonful of her (again ingenious) Almond Whip (see the recipe for Summer Fruit Parfait, page 256).

Serves 4 to 6

Ⓥ Vegan

3 cups almond milk (or your favorite
    nondairy milk)
1½ tablespoons arrowroot
⅔ cup good-quality maple syrup
A pinch of fine sea salt
3 tablespoons agar flakes
4 ounces unsweetened chocolate
1 teaspoon pure vanilla extract

In a small bowl, pour 3 tablespoons of the almond milk over the arrowroot, stir to dissolve, and set aside.

Pour the remaining almond milk, the maple syrup, and the salt into a small pot and sprinkle the agar flakes over the surface; let stand 15 minutes to soften. Meanwhile, chop the chocolate into small pieces and set it aside.

Over medium-low heat, slowly bring the milk mixture to a boil. Lower the heat slightly and stir continuously until all the agar is dissolved, about 2 minutes. Stir in the arrowroot mixture and cook, stirring, until the mixture is thickened.

Turn off the heat and whisk the chopped chocolate and vanilla into the milk mixture until smooth. Pour the pudding into a bowl and place it, uncovered, in the refrigerator until it's completely cool, about 1 hour.

Remove the cooled pudding from the refrigerator and spoon it into a blender or food processor. Blend or process, stopping to scrape down the sides, until the pudding is wonderfully smooth. Transfer the pudding into dessert cups and chill until ready to serve.

DARLEEN'S CHEESECAKE

A decadent, classic dessert made gloriously good for you. Darleen recommends eating this with fresh fruit. We especially love it with slices of ripe, sweet summertime peaches.

Serves 12

V Vegan

FOR THE CRUST
Cooking spray
1½ cups almond meal
¼ teaspoon fine sea salt
3 tablespoons coconut oil, melted
2 tablespoons maple sugar or coconut sugar

FOR THE FILLING
A 14-ounce package sprouted silken tofu
 (Darleen recommends the Wildwood brand)
1 cup almond meal
¼ cup brown rice syrup
⅓ cup grade A light maple syrup
1 tablespoon sweet white miso paste
¼ cup tapioca starch or arrowroot
¼ teaspoon fine salt
2 teaspoons pure vanilla extract
¾ teaspoon almond extract
Zest of ½ lemon

Preheat the oven to 350°F and coat an 8-inch springform pan with cooking spray.

Mix together all the crust ingredients and press the mixture into the bottom of the prepared pan, making sure it's even and there are no cracks. Pressing the mixture down with the back of a large spoon helps.

Bake the crust until lightly browned, 10 to 15 minutes, and set it aside to cool.

Meanwhile, place the tofu in a colander to drain, then transfer to the bowl of a food processor or blender with the remaining filling ingredients and process or blend to a uniform creamy consistency.

Pour the filling over the cooled crust and use a rubber spatula to smooth the top.

Place the pan in a baking dish with sides at least 2 inches high. Place the whole thing on the middle rack of the oven and carefully pour the contents of a kettle of boiling water into the baking dish so it comes halfway up the sides of the cheesecake pan. Bake the cheesecake until the center is no longer liquidy and the top is a light golden brown, 1 to 1¼ hours. Carefully remove the cheesecake from the water bath, let it cool to room temperature, then refrigerate for at least 2 hours before serving.

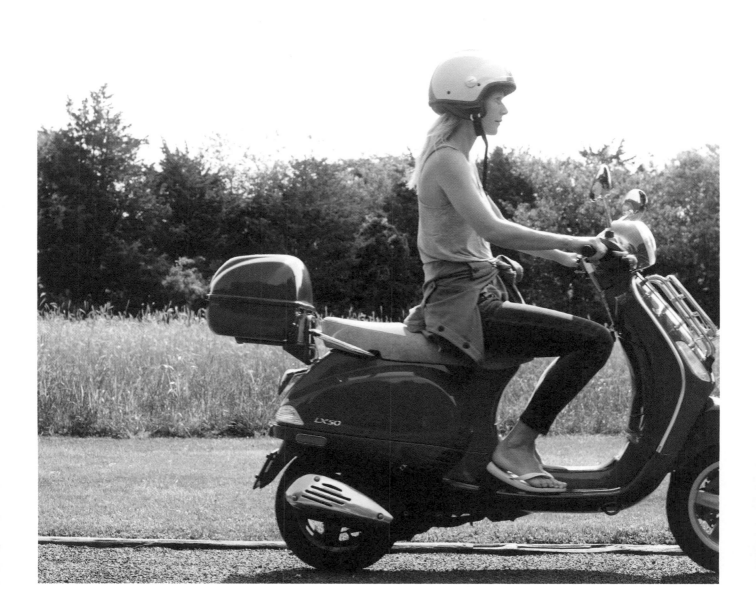

BASIC RECIPES

These recipes are for simple basics that are good to have on hand to really build flavor into any dish. When you're eating clean, using great sauces and stocks is the key to making sure you don't feel deprived. And when your senses are satisfied with lots of deep, delicious flavor, you'll never realize that you're eliminating anything from your diet.

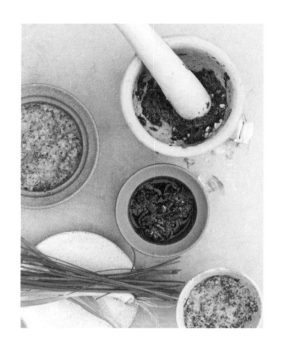
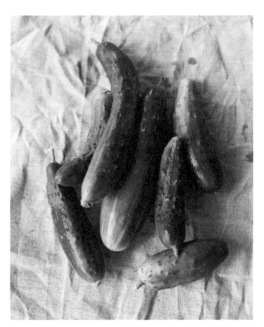
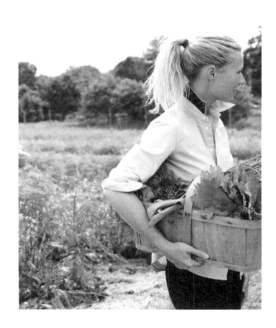
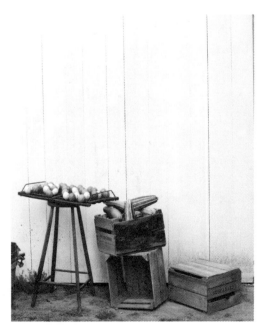

CHICKEN STOCK

This straightforward chicken stock is foolproof and makes a great base. Be sure to use organic chicken!

Makes about 10 cups

Ⓔ Elimination Diet

1 whole 3- to 4-pound organic chicken, washed
1 teaspoon black peppercorns
1 bay leaf
2 stalks celery, roughly chopped
1 large onion, peeled and roughly chopped
2 carrots, peeled and roughly chopped
3 sprigs of parsley
3 sprigs of thyme
1 teaspoon coarse sea salt

Put all the ingredients into a large soup pot, cover with cold water (it should take about 3 quarts), and bring to a boil over high heat. Skim any foam that rises to the top, turn the heat to low, and simmer for 1½ hours. Let the stock cool, then strain into containers to freeze for up to 6 months. Discard the cooked aromatics—their flavor will be spent at this point. The cooked chicken makes great chicken salad, or you can shred it into the strained broth, add a couple of fresh carrots cut into coins and some diced celery, and enjoy some delicious soup.

VEGETABLE STOCK

As vegetable stock out of a box can be completely uninspired, I started making and freezing this robust stock. It brings vegetarian soups up a notch.

Makes 12 cups

Ⓔ Elimination Diet Ⓥ Vegan

1 large yellow onion, peeled and roughly chopped
2 large carrots, peeled and roughly chopped
1 stalk celery, roughly chopped
1 large leek, thoroughly washed and roughly chopped
3 garlic cloves, peeled and whacked with the side of your knife
4 sprigs of Italian parsley
4 sprigs of fresh thyme
2 sprigs of fresh tarragon
1 bay leaf
1 teaspoon coarse salt
1 teaspoon black peppercorns
3 quarts cold water

Combine everything in a pot. Bring to a boil, lower the heat, and simmer for 45 minutes. Let the stock cool and strain into a clean container. Discard the solids. Keeps for a week in an airtight container in the refrigerator or for 6 months in the freezer.

GO-TO TOMATO SAUCE

This recipe makes a simple, perfect tomato sauce. Slow-cooked to bring out the sweetness, it is the perfect base for many of the dishes in this book.

Makes 4 cups

Ⓥ Vegan

2 tablespoons extra virgin olive oil
6 garlic cloves, thinly sliced
4 large fresh basil leaves
Two 28-ounce cans whole peeled tomatoes with
    their juice
Coarse sea salt
Freshly ground black pepper

Heat the olive oil in a large saucepan over low heat, add the garlic, and cook for 5 minutes. Add 2 of the basil leaves and stir for 1 minute. Add the tomatoes with their juice and the 2 remaining basil leaves. Turn the heat to high. Bring the sauce to a boil, turn the heat to low, season with salt and pepper, and let it bubble away on low heat for 45 minutes, stirring occasionally and crushing the tomatoes with a wooden spoon. Cool and refrigerate. This sauce keeps for a week in an airtight container in the refrigerator, or for 6 months in the freezer.

LEE'S SRIRACHA

One day when I was talking to my friend Lee Gross about my love for this spicy, smoky bottled condiment, he informed me that it was full of chemicals. Luckily, he came up with this version, which is just as delicious and preservative free! Don't worry—it still keeps for ages in the fridge.

Makes 5 cups

(V) Vegan (substitute soy sauce for the fish sauce)

1¼ cups peeled garlic cloves
1 pound red jalapeños, stemmed and sliced
    into thin rings (for a milder sauce,
    remove some seeds)
2¼ cups rice wine vinegar
¼ cup plus 1 tablespoon brown rice syrup
2 tablespoons coarse sea salt
1 tablespoon arrowroot
2 tablespoons fish sauce (or soy sauce)

Put the garlic cloves in a small saucepan and add cold water just to cover. Bring to a boil, immediately drain, cool the garlic under running water, and return it to the saucepan. Cover with cold water and repeat the blanching process. Thinly slice the blanched garlic and combine with the jalapeños and vinegar in a larger pot. Bring to a boil, cook for 3 minutes, and remove from the heat. Add the brown rice syrup and salt and stir to combine. Let the mixture sit undisturbed for 1 hour to steep and cool.

Whiz the mixture in a powerful blender until smooth (it's okay if all the seeds don't blend in). Return the pureed sauce to the pot, bring to a boil, lower the heat, and simmer for 10 to 15 minutes, skimming off any foam, until the sauce is slightly reduced and has some body.

In a small bowl, dissolve the arrowroot with 1 tablespoon of lukewarm water. Whisk into the simmering sauce and cook for 2 minutes more, or until the sauce is nicely thickened (it should be slightly thinner than ketchup). Remove the sauce from the heat, let it cool slightly, and stir in the fish sauce. Store in a screw-top jar or bottle in the refrigerator for up to 6 months.

LEE'S HOISIN SAUCE

We use this in so many dishes we can't remember life before it.

Makes about 1 cup

Ⓥ Vegan

1 tablespoon neutral oil (like canola, grapeseed, or safflower oil)
1 large garlic clove, minced
½ teaspoon Chinese five-spice powder
½ cup red miso paste
½ cup good-quality maple syrup
2 tablespoons brown rice vinegar

Heat the oil in a small saucepan over medium heat. Add the garlic and five-spice powder and cook for about 30 seconds, or until wonderfully fragrant. Whisk in the remaining ingredients, bring to a boil, and cook, whisking or stirring constantly, for 3 to 4 minutes, or until slightly thickened. Let the sauce cool before using. It keeps well in the refrigerator for a few days.

GO-TO BLACK BEANS

By adding a few aromatics to a can of black beans, you get that Mexican restaurant flavor without hours of soaking and cooking.

Serves 4 as a side dish

Ⓔ Elimination Diet Ⓥ Vegan Ⓟ Protein-Packed

2 tablespoons extra virgin olive oil
1 garlic clove, finely chopped
A 15½-ounce can black beans
4 sprigs of cilantro
A pinch of coarse sea salt

Heat the olive oil in a small pot set over medium heat. Add the garlic and cook, stirring, just until fragrant, 1 or 2 minutes. Add the entire can of beans (including the liquid), the cilantro, and the salt and turn the heat to high. Once the beans begin to boil, turn the heat to low and simmer until the beans have lost their tin can flavor and aren't too watery, about 15 minutes. Remove the cilantro before serving.

LEE'S PONZU

This mixture is lovely on grilled fish and vegetables. If you can't find prepared ponzu to doctor as Lee does, simply substitute ⅓ cup soy sauce, ½ cup bottled yuzu or fresh lime juice, and ¼ cup mirin. You can also turn this into a vinaigrette—which is delicious on any salad, especially ones with avocado—by whisking in 2 tablespoons of toasted sesame oil.

Makes a generous cup

Ⓥ Vegan

2 large strips of zest from an orange
Juice of 1 orange
4 garlic cloves, peeled and crushed
10 quarter-sized coins of peeled ginger, crushed
1⅓ cups prepared ponzu sauce without any MSG
    (check in your local Asian grocery store or
    asianfoodgrocer.com)

Combine all of the ingredients in a small saucepan set over high heat. Bring to a boil, lower the heat, and simmer over a low flame for 10 minutes. Turn off the heat, let the dressing cool and strain before using.

SOAKED RAW ALMONDS

E Elimination Diet **V** Vegan **P** Protein-Packed

We all know how healthy and nutritious almonds are for us—they're full of omegas, protein, magnesium, vitamin E, and zinc. But all that great stuff is actually really hard to benefit from because almonds have an enzyme in their coating that makes them difficult to digest. The harder anything is to digest, the more work your body has to do to get to all the nutrients and the more you miss out. Good news though! If you simply soak raw almonds in plenty of water for at least half a day, the enzyme will break down and you're good to go. We keep raw almonds in a container of fresh water in the fridge for up to a week for snacks and smoothies (see the Almond + Kale smoothie on page 207).

SOAKED GOJI BERRIES

E Elimination Diet **V** Vegan

Goji berries have been considered a miracle food for ages and have long been incorporated in treatments for high blood pressure and diabetes, and to improve brain health. Like any berry, goji berries are super-packed with antioxidants, those wonderful compounds that help bolster the immune system and keep us from getting sick and aging rapidly. Because they're incredibly rich in vitamin A, goji berries are also said to be really great for protecting vision. Basically, they're pretty amazing. I pop dried ones like potato chips and also soak them overnight in water to soften them so I can easily blend them into smoothies, like the Red Smoothie (see page 208) or the Kid Smoothie (see page 224).

AN EGG, THREE WAYS

Serve 1 or 2 eggs per person

Ⓟ Protein-Packed

Loaded with omegas and vitamins, eggs make for a perfect high-protein meal or snack. Here are three ways to cook an egg perfectly.

A POACHED EGG

Coarse sea salt
1 teaspoon white wine vinegar
1 fresh organic egg

Boil a saucepan of water, turn the heat to low, and let the water relax to a simmer. Add a large pinch of salt and the vinegar to the water. Crack the egg into a ramekin or small bowl and stir the water gently with a wooden spoon to create a whirlpool. Carefully slip the egg into the center of the whirlpool and poach until cooked to your liking. I find that 3 minutes yields a perfectly poached egg with a slightly runny center. Remove the egg with a slotted spoon, blot dry on a paper towel, and serve immediately.

A HARD-BOILED EGG

1 fresh organic egg

Place your egg in a saucepan of cold water and set it over high heat. Once the water comes to a boil, cover the pot and turn off the heat. Let the egg sit for exactly 6 minutes if you like the yolk just barely cooked through, 7 if you like it quite firm but not dried out. Transfer the egg into a bowl of ice water to stop it from cooking. Carefully peel off and discard the shell. (Curiously, the older the egg, the easier it is to peel.)

AN OLIVE OIL–FRIED EGG

2 tablespoons extra virgin olive oil
1 organic egg
Coarse sea salt

Heat the olive oil in a small nonstick skillet or griddle pan set over high heat. Crack the egg right into the hot oil and sprinkle with a bit of coarse salt. Cover the skillet and cook for just 1 minute, or until the white is cooked through and the yolk is just set (or for 1 more minute if you prefer your egg more well done). Slip the egg from the pan onto a plate, a slice of gluten-free toast, a bowl of quinoa, or a bowl of stir-fried vegetables—anywhere!

ORANGE MARMALADE

We used to use store-bought orange marmalade as the sweet secret ingredient in Korean Barbecue Sauce (see page 283). We set out to see if we could successfully make our own, without any sugar, and it turns out the homemade version is not just great as a backbone for any barbecue sauce, it's also wonderful anywhere you'd normally use jam. You can substitute any citrus here—Meyer lemons, grapefruit…they all work nicely.

Makes nearly 3 cups

Ⓥ Vegan

3 navel oranges, stem ends trimmed off
    and discarded
Juice of 1 lemon
2 cups water
1 cup xylitol or good raw honey

Cut the oranges in half. Scoop the insides—the flesh, juice, and seeds—into a food processor and reserve the skins. Puree the insides until smooth and pour into a heavy-bottomed saucepan. Slice the skins into matchsticks and add them to the saucepan along with the lemon juice and the water. Turn the heat to high and bring the mixture to a boil. Lower the heat and simmer for 1½ hours, uncovered, or until the rinds are very, very soft. Add the xylitol or honey and turn the heat back to high. Boil the marmalade, stirring quite often, for 10 minutes, or until the marmalade begins to pull away from the sides of the pan. Turn off the heat and let the marmalade cool before transferring to a jar. Keeps in the fridge for up to a month.

PICKLED JALAPEÑOS

Every year I grow jalapeños in our vegetable garden at the beach. Last year there were so many that we pickled them, and now we can enjoy them on salads, sandwiches, and tacos all year.

Makes 1 Vegenaise jar's worth of pickles

Ⓥ Vegan

¾ cup white wine vinegar
¾ cup water
1 tablespoon coarse sea salt
A pinch of celery seed
1 teaspoon coriander seeds
1 teaspoon black peppercorns
8 large jalapeños, thinly sliced
1 bay leaf
1 garlic clove, thinly sliced

Combine the vinegar, water, salt, celery seed, coriander seeds, and peppercorns in a small saucepan over high heat, bring to a boil, and turn off the heat. Meanwhile, pack your empty Vegenaise jar with the jalapeños and stuff the bay leaf and the garlic slices in and among the peppers. Pour the vinegar mixture over the jalapeños, being sure to get all the seeds into the mix. The liquid should completely cover the peppers. Let the jar cool to room temperature, then tightly screw on the lid and stash the jar in the fridge. The peppers are good to go after a week, but they keep up to a year in the refrigerator—seriously!

BREAD + BUTTER PICKLES

Bread-and-butter pickles were impossible to find in the UK, so we set about creating our own delicious version. And ours are sugar free!

Makes about 1 pint

Ⓥ Vegan

1 pound cucumbers, ends trimmed, sliced into coins (the smaller the cucumbers you can find, the better; we like Kirby and Israeli cucumbers best—it will take about 6 of these small guys to yield 1 pound)
1 small yellow onion, thinly sliced
2 tablespoons coarse sea salt
½ cup white wine vinegar
½ cup xylitol or raw honey
1 teaspoon coriander seeds
1 teaspoon black mustard seeds
½ teaspoon ground turmeric
½ teaspoon black peppercorns
A pinch of celery seed
1 bay leaf

Combine the cucumbers, onion, and salt in a large mixing bowl of very icy ice water and let them sit for 2 hours (this will help keep the pickles very crunchy).

Meanwhile, bring the vinegar, xylitol or honey, and seasonings to a boil in a large pot. Drain the cucumbers and onions and add them to the pot. Bring back to a boil, immediately turn off the heat, and transfer the entire mixture to a glass jar. Once the jar cools to room temperature, put a lid on it and store in the refrigerator for up to a month (though the pickles rarely last that long!).

SUPER-SPICY TOMATILLO SALSA

This recipe is a little labor-intensive, but it's totally worth it, since this salsa has remarkable flavor with zero fat, gluten, dairy, or sugar. It's amazing to consider how something made completely out of produce can pack this much of a punch.

Makes 1 pint

Ⓥ Vegan

1 poblano pepper
6 tomatilloes, papery layers and stems discarded, roughly chopped
2 jalapeños, stems discarded, roughly chopped (seeds and all—or seed the peppers or use less if you're not a hothead)
½ white onion, peeled and thinly sliced
A small handful of cilantro
Juice of 1 lime
1 tablespoon Pickled Jalapeños (see page 280)
Coarse sea salt

Roast the poblano pepper over an open gas flame on medium-high, rotating now and then with tongs, until it's charred all over. If you have an electric stove, it's best to broil the pepper, but set your oven rack in the middle of the oven so it takes the pepper a bit of time to char. Be patient; you want to not only blacken the skin, but soften the pepper, too—it should take a good 15 minutes. Place the pepper in a bowl and cover it tightly with plastic wrap or place it in a paper bag (both methods help create steam which will help you get the skin off). Once it's cool enough to handle, slip off and discard the charred skin, the stem, and the seeds. You don't have to be too careful about the peeling; a little char is okay in the final salsa. Set the pepper aside.

Preheat the broiler and line a sheet pan with tinfoil. Combine the tomatilloes with 1 of the chopped jalapeños and the onion on the prepared sheet pan. Broil the vegetables, stirring now and then, until collapsed and a bit charred, about 10 minutes.

Transfer the broiled vegetables to a food processor along with the poblano, the remaining raw jalapeño, the cilantro, the lime juice, and the pickled jalapeños. Puree everything and season to taste with salt.

ROASTED TOMATO + CHIPOTLE SALSA

This easy flavor-packed salsa livens up grilled fish and tacos and is perfect with gluten-free tortilla chips. Also, they say roasting tomatoes lowers their acidity...

Makes 1 cup

V Vegan

4 vine-ripened tomatoes, cores removed, roughly chopped
1 small yellow onion, roughly chopped
1 tablespoon extra virgin olive oil
1 chipotle pepper (or more or less, depending on your heat tolerance—a whole pepper makes this salsa quite hot!) from a can of chipotles packed in adobo sauce
3 tablespoons cilantro
2 tablespoons freshly squeezed lime juice
Coarse sea salt

Preheat the broiler to high, placing the rack in the upper third of the oven. Line a baking sheet with tinfoil and toss, directly on the sheet, the tomatoes and onion with the olive oil. Broil, stirring now and then, until the tomatoes have collapsed and the onions have softened a bit and everything is slightly charred, about 10 minutes. Place the tomatoes and onions in a food processor with the chipotle, cilantro, and lime juice and blitz until everything is pureed. Remove the salsa to a bowl and season to taste with salt.

KOREAN SALSA

Following the same technique as for the Roasted Tomato + Chipotle Salsa, the Korean flavors in this version yield a sauce that's vital to Korean Chicken Tacos (see page 116). It's also delicious on eggs or any kind of grilled protein (try it with the Grilled Steak, instead of the Melted Anchovies + Rosemary, on page 120, or with a piece of salmon).

Makes 1 cup

1½ cups cherry tomatoes, halved
1 small yellow onion, roughly chopped
1 tablespoon extra virgin olive oil
2 tablespoons gochujang (Korean red pepper paste, available at Asian markets or Hmart.com)
1 garlic clove, minced
1 teaspoon fish sauce

Preheat the broiler to high, placing the rack in the upper third of the oven. Line a baking sheet with tinfoil and toss, directly on the sheet, the tomatoes and onion with the olive oil. Broil, stirring now and then, until the tomatoes have collapsed and the onions have softened a bit and everything is slightly charred, about 10 minutes. Place the tomatoes and onions in a food processor with the remaining ingredients and blitz until pureed. Remove the salsa to a bowl and season to taste with salt.

KOREAN BARBECUE SAUCE

This easy sauce depends on the unexpected combination of orange and chili. An essential component of Korean Chicken Tacos (see page 116), this barbecue sauce can also go on top of any cooked protein and is really good dabbed on roasted sweet potatoes.

Makes 1 cup

½ cup Orange Marmalade (see page 279)
¼ cup gochujang (Korean red pepper paste, available at Asian markets or Hmart.com)
1 teaspoon soy sauce
1 teaspoon toasted sesame oil
1 teaspoon fish sauce
1 garlic clove, minced

Puree all the ingredients in a blender.

SRIRACHA MAYO

This requires just a stir to make, but it's a flavor bomb and is so delicious alongside Salmon Burgers with Pickled Ginger + Coriander (see page 128).

Makes ⅔ cup

Ⓥ Vegan

½ cup Vegenaise
1 tablespoon good-quality maple syrup or raw honey
1 tablespoon Lee's Sriracha (see page 274)
2 tablespoons freshly squeezed lime juice
Coarse sea salt

Whisk everything together.

CHIMICHURRI

Basically the South American equivalent of pesto, chimichurri normally accompanies grilled red meat, but we think its punchy, slightly spicy flavor is totally at home with vegetables (try the Sautéed Corn with Chimichurri on page 170), on roasted or grilled fish or chicken, or even stirred into cooked brown rice or quinoa. It's a good condiment to have on hand.

Makes ½ cup

E Elimination Diet **V** Vegan

1 packed cup Italian parsley
½ packed cup cilantro
2 garlic cloves, finely minced
1 jalapeño, seeded and finely minced
½ cup extra virgin olive oil
3 tablespoons red wine vinegar
½ teaspoon ground cumin
1 teaspoon coarse sea salt

Pulse everything together in a food processor. Let it sit for at least 20 minutes before serving.

SALSA VERDE

Salsa Verde is one of my favorite salsas/dressings/dips. It's always fresh and delicious, and you can substitute whatever herbs you have handy. I love it slathered on grilled fish or as a condiment for raw veggies.

Makes nearly 1 cup

E Elimination Diet

2 garlic cloves, minced
Coarse salt
4 good-quality anchovy fillets
A dozen basil leaves, chopped
¼ cup chopped Italian parsley
2 handfuls of arugula, chopped
1 teaspoon red wine vinegar
⅓ cup extra virgin olive oil
Freshly ground black pepper

With a mortar and pestle, mash the garlic and a pinch of salt into a paste. Add the anchovies and crush with the pestle. Add the herbs and arugula and crush them into the garlic and anchovy mixture (but don't go overboard—it's nice to leave this rough and rustic). Stir in the red wine vinegar and olive oil with a spoon. Season to taste with pepper and more salt if needed. Let the Salsa Verde sit for at least 20 minutes before serving. While you can definitely make it early in the day, be sure to eat it on the same day you make it, or it tends to lose its bright flavor.

CLASSIC PESTO

Pesto is always a crowd-pleaser. In this version we cut out the Parmesan for an extra-healthy preparation without sacrificing flavor.

Makes ½ cup

E Elimination Diet **V** Vegan

3 tablespoons pine nuts
1 garlic clove, finely minced
1 packed cup basil leaves
¼ cup extra virgin olive oil
½ teaspoon coarse sea salt

Combine the nuts and garlic in the bowl of a food processor and pulse until the nuts are finely ground. Add the basil and pulse a few times, until it's roughly chopped. Add the olive oil and salt and pulse a few more times, until the pesto is just combined but still has a slightly rough texture.

SCALLION + MINT PESTO

A variation on a classic basil pesto, this dairy-free version relies on the scallions and mint to give it zing.

Makes 1 cup

E Elimination Diet **V** Vegan

½ cup toasted almonds
2 small garlic cloves, minced
A dozen scallions, white and light green
        parts only, roughly chopped
⅓ cup mint leaves
⅓ cup extra virgin olive oil
⅓ cup water
2 teaspoons freshly squeezed lemon juice
1½ teaspoons coarse sea salt

Puree everything in a powerful blender until smooth.

PUMPKIN SEED PESTO

This is delicious as a dip for veggies or tossed with rice noodles.

Makes nearly 1 cup

E Elimination Diet **V** Vegan

½ cup toasted pumpkin seeds (toast on a
    sheet pan in a 400°F oven for 5 minutes
    and let cool)
1 garlic clove, minced
2 teaspoons capers
1 tablespoon chopped chives
Leaves from 2 sprigs of Italian parsley
4 large leaves of basil
¼ cup freshly squeezed lemon juice
2 tablespoons extra virgin olive oil
⅓ cup water
⅓ teaspoon coarse sea salt

Combine all the ingredients in a blender and blitz until completely pureed.

SPICY CASHEW MOMENT

It's hard to say exactly what this is. Inspired by the smoked cashew salsa at a great Mexican restaurant in Manhattan's West Village called Empellón, this condiment is also an homage to all the rich cashew blends beloved by vegans and raw foodists, bless their hippie hearts. This tastes, truly, like nacho cheese. It's got an unbelievably creamy, rich texture. We like it on tortilla chips or on seeded crackers, and we dollop it wherever we would use sour cream. A spoonful is especially good on top of a bowl of Turkey + Black Bean Chili with Sweet Potatoes (see page 106).

Makes 1 cup

V Vegan **P** Protein-Packed

2 tablespoons extra virgin olive oil
1 cup raw cashews
½ teaspoon ground cumin
½ teaspoon ground chili powder
½ teaspoon sweet pimentón
½ jalapeño, seeded and chopped (add more or
        less, depending on your taste; we find
        ½ pepper is on the border of spicy without
        being overpowering)
3 tablespoons freshly squeezed lime juice
⅓ cup extra virgin olive oil
⅓ cup water
1 teaspoon coarse sea salt

Heat the olive oil in a small skillet over medium-high heat. Add the cashews, sprinkle them with the cumin, chili powder, and pimentón, and cook, stirring now and then, until the spices are toasted and the nuts are just beginning to turn brown, about 2 minutes. Transfer the cashews to a high-powered blender along with the rest of the ingredients and blend until completely smooth and creamy.

SEAWEED SESAME SPRINKLE

For a little salty, crunchy Eden Shake kind of condiment make this. It adds texture and tremendous flavor to Steamed Fish with Soy + Spicy Sesame Oil (see page 137) and is also amazing on A Plain Roasted Sweet Potato (see page 152) or on Avocado Toast (see page 34).

Makes ¼ cup

E Elimination Diet **V** Vegan

3 sheets toasted nori seaweed
2 tablespoons toasted sesame seeds (white and
        black seeds both work)
A large pinch of coarse sea salt

Break the nori into small pieces and grind the pieces in a coffee grinder until they're powdery. Transfer the nori to a small bowl and thoroughly combine it with the sesame seeds and salt.

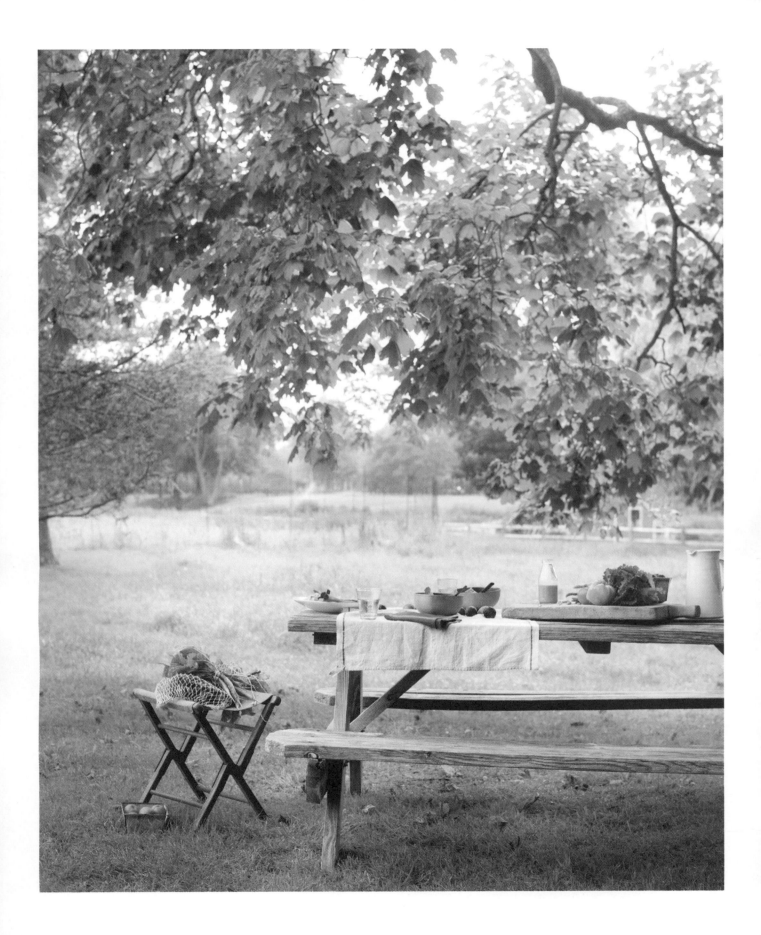

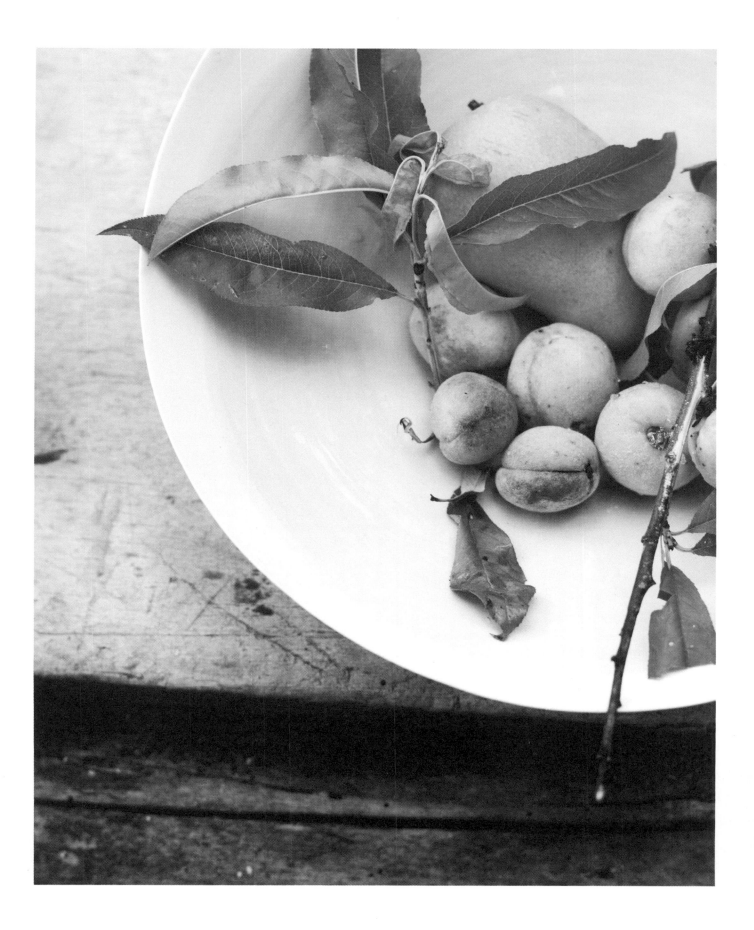

A BODY BUILDER WEEK

	Breakfast	Post-workout snack	Lunch	Afternoon Snack	Dinner
Monday	An Actully Good Egg-White Omelet, Huevos Rancheros version (see page 50)	Bernardo's Pumpkin Pie Shake (see page 209)	Lee's Chopped Vietnamese Salad (see page 58) with grilled fish	a handful of Soaked Raw Almonds (see page 277)	Middle Eastern Turkey Burgers (see page 108; skip the yogurt sauce) with grilled asparagus
Tuesday	Leftover Quinoa either way (see page 33)	Body Builder Smoothie (see page 209)	Turkey + Black Bean Chili with Sweet Potatoes (see page 106)	A Plain Roasted Sweet Potato (see page 152)	Grilled Steak (without the Melted Anchovies + Rosemary; see page 120) and a nice arugula salad dressed with lots of lemon
Wednesday	Egg-White Omelet, Spinach + Mushroom version (see page 51) with Roasted Tomato + Chipotle Salsa (see page 282)	Bernardo's Pumpkin Pie Shake (see page 209)	Steamed Fish with Soy + Spicy Sesame Oil (see page 137), with A Plain Roasted Sweet Potato (see page 152)	Kale Chips (see page 246; make without salt)	Perfect Herbed Grilled Chicken (see page 100) and steamed green beans with plenty of lemon
Thursday	Power Oatmeal (see page 34)	Body Builder Smoothie (see page 209) with some frozen blueberries thrown in	Chicken Burger, Thai Style (see page 111) with Asian Greens with Garlic, Ginger + Fish Sauce (see page 162) and Perfectly Cooked Quinoa (see page 178)	A Plain Roasted Sweet Potato (see page 152)	Many-Mushroom Soup (see page 81) with Grilled Salmon with Grilled Lemon Vinaigrette (see page 143) and steamed spinach
Friday	Egg-White Omelet, Spinach + Mushroom version (see page 51)	Bernardo's Pumpkin Pie Shake (see page 209)	Spicy Sweet Potato Soup with Chipotle + Coriander (see page 88), along with a big green salad and Perfect Herbed Grilled Chicken (see page 100)	a handful of Soaked Raw Almonds (see page 277)	Turkey Meatballs (see page 105) with steamed broccoli
Saturday	Leftover Quinoa either way (see page 33)	Body Builder Smoothie (see page 209) with a tablespoon of raw cacao added	Salmon Burger with Pickled Ginger + Coriander (see page 128), with steamed snap peas and Perfectly Cooked Brown Rice (see page 178)	A Plain Roasted Sweet Potato (see page 152)	Grilled Striped Bass with Cucumber + Clementine Salsa (see page 140) alongside Super-Healthy Kosheri (see page 179)
Sunday	Have a day off! Life's too short!				

A DETOX WEEK

	Breakfast Drink	Morning snack	Lunch	Afternoon Drink	Dinner
Monday	The Best Green Juice (see page 212)	a handful of Soaked Raw Almonds (see page 277)	Beet Greens Soup (see page 89)	Beet, Carrot, Apple + Ginger Juice (see page 213)	Barbecued Chicken, Spanish Style (see page 97) with roasted asparagus
Tuesday	The Best Green Juice (see page 212)	a nice pear	Arugula Salad with Roasted Beets, Squash + Shallots with Apple Cider Vinaigrette (see page 69) along with Perfectly Cooked Quinoa (see page 178)	Creamy Avocado + Cacao Smoothie (see page 208)	Miso Soup with Watercress (see page 78), Fish Roasted in Salt, Thai Style (see page 134), and Asian Greens with Garlic, Ginger + Fish Sauce (see page 162)
Wednesday	The Best Green Juice (see page 212)	Kale Chips (see page 246)	Millet "Falafel" with Avocado Relish (see page 203; skip the tomatoes)	Cucumber, Basil + Lime Juice (see page 213)	Lee's Braised Daikon (see page 164) and Steamed Fish with Soy + Spicy Sesame Oil (see page 137)
Thursday	The Best Green Juice (see page 212)	a handful of Soaked Raw Almonds (see page 277)	Chicken Burger, Thai Style (see page 111) with Korean Slaw (see page 161)	Red Smoothie (see page 208; make it without the yogurt and substitute extra raspberries for the strawberries)	Broccoli + Arugula Soup (see page 78) and Turkey Meatballs (see page 105; skip the tomato sauce) with an arugula salad
Friday	The Best Green Juice (see page 212)	an apple with a spoonful of almond butter	Lee's Chopped Vietnamese Salad (see page 58) and Grilled Salmon with Grilled Lemon Vinaigrette (see page 143)	Beet, Carrot, Apple + Ginger Juice (see page 213)	Braised Chicken with Green Olives + Lemon (see page 98) and Broccoli Rabe with Garlic + Red Chili (see page 154)
Saturday	The Best Green Juice (see page 212)	Homemade Almond Milk/Horchata (see page 220)	Spinach with Miso-Almond Sauce (see page 162) with Perfectly Cooked Brown Rice (see page 178)	Almond + Kale Smoothie (see page 207)	Grilled Salmon with Grilled Lemon Vinaigrette (see page 143) along with Super-Healthy Kosheri (see page 179)
Sunday	The Best Green Juice (see page 212)	a bowl of blueberries and raspberries	Brown Rice Pasta with Tuna, Olives, Fried Capers + Parsley (see page 192; make it without the tuna)	Bernardo's Pumpkin Pie Shake (see page 209)	grilled fish and steamed artichokes with Salsa Verde (see page 284)

A FAMILY-FRIENDLY WEEK

	Breakfast	Lunch	Dinner
Monday	a batch of Sweet Potato + Five-Spice Muffins (see page 41)	Healthy Tuna Salad (see page 129) on toasted gluten-free English muffins	Chicken Fajitas (see page 237) with all the fixings
Tuesday	Scrambled Tofu (see page 47) with sliced avocado and Go-To Black Beans (see page 275)	Best Roasted Turkey Breast (see page 109) wrapped in lettuce with turkey bacon and Vegenaise	Veggie Dumplings (see page 228) and Rice Cream Sundaes (see page 242)
Wednesday	a batch of Banana-Date Muffins (see page 46)	Chinese Chicken Salad (see page 71; leave the components plain for the kids)	Crazy Good Fish Tacos (see page 144) with all the fixings
Thursday	Power Oatmeal (see page 34)	Avocado Toast (see page 34) and Chicken Soup with Kale + Carrots (see page 82)	Teriyaki Chicken (see page 96) with Asian Greens with Garlic, Ginger + Fish Sauce (see page 162) and Roasted Carrots with Honey + Soy Sauce (see page 232)
Friday	Design your own smoothies! Set out a bunch of ingredients as per the smoothies on pages 207 to 209 and let everyone customize	gluten-free toast with hummus and Scallion + Mint Pesto (see page 285) and NY Street Vendor Salad with Yogurt-Tahini Dressing (see page 62)	Chicken + White Bean Chili (see page 102) and Bibb lettuce with Green Goddess Dressing (see page 75)
Saturday	Buckwheat + Banana Pancakes (see page 42)	Tandoori Turkey Kabobs (see page 107) with Super-Healthy Kosheri (see page 179)	Best Gluten-Free Fish Fingers either way (see page 234), with corn on the cob and iceberg wedge with tomatoes and Old Bay Ranch Dressing (see page 75)
Sunday	"Buttermilk" Waffles (see page 38) with turkey bacon	Korean Chicken Tacos (see page 116) with all the fixings	Turkey Meatballs (see page 105) with brown rice pasta and steamed broccoli

A VEGAN WEEK

	Breakfast	Lunch	Dinner
Monday	Scrambled Tofu (see page 47) with sliced avocado and Go-To Black Beans (see page 275)	Japanese Restaurant–Style Salad with Carrot-Ginger Dressing (see page 65) and plenty of avocado	Roasted Cauliflower + Chickpeas with Mustard + Parsley (see page 173), Beet Salad with Scallion + Mint Pesto (see page 155), and Roasted Leeks either way (see page 175)
Tuesday	"Buttermilk" Waffles (see page 38) with fresh berries	Millet "Falafel" with Avocado + Tomato Relish (see page 203)	Beet, Fennel + Apple Soup (see page 79) and Polenta with Shiitakes + Fried Leeks (see page 188)
Wednesday	a batch of Millet-Fig Muffins (see page 43)	Grilled Asparagus + Portobellos with Shallot + Soy Dressing (see page 152) with Perfectly Cooked Brown Rice (see page 178) and some kimchi	Scallion Pancakes with Brown Rice Flour (see page 189), Black Rice with Fresh Coconut (see page 183), and Grilled Eggplant with Ginger, Chili + Cilantro (see page 166)
Thursday	Quinoa Granola with Olive Oil + Maple Syrup (see page 30), with Homemade Almond Milk/Horchata (see page 220) and fresh blueberries	Quinoa with Butternut Squash, Scallions + Parsley (see page 200) and Roasted Romanesco with Aioli + Fried Capers (see page 174)	Turkey + Black Bean Chili with Sweet Potatoes (see page 106) with Spicy Cashew Moment (see page 286) and a green salad with Mexican Green Goddess Dressing (see page 57)
Friday	Leftover Quinoa, Way Two (see page 33)	Power Chopped Salad with Creamy Parsley Dressing minus the hard-boiled egg (see page 61)	Risotto with Peas + Greens (see page 180) and a nice green salad
Saturday	Buckwheat + Banana Pancakes with maple syrup (see page 42)	Quinoa with Mushrooms + Arugula (see page 200) and any one of the Three Simple Beet Salads (see page 155)	Go-To Black Beans (see page 275) with Mexican Tomato Rice (see page 183) and Mango + Avocado Salad with Balsamic-Lime Vinaigrette (see page 68)
Sunday	Avocado Toast (see page 34)	Baked Beans with Maple + Molasses (see page 167), Charred Corn with Sage (see page 170), and a tomato salad	Buckwheat Soba Noodles with Ginger-Scallion Broth (see page 199), Asparagus with Miso-Almond Sauce (see page 162), and Lee's Braised Daikon (see page 164)

JUST GREAT, HEALTHY, EVERYDAY EATING

	Breakfast	Lunch	Afternoon Snack	Dinner
Monday	Avocado Toast (see page 34) and The Best Green Juice (see page 212)	Frankies-esque Beet Salad (see page 155) and Middle Eastern Turkey Burgers with Cucumber + Yogurt Sauce (see page 108)	raw veggies with Green Goddess Dressing (see page 75)	Two-Pan Chicken (Korean style; see the recipe for Two-Pan Chicken with Harissa, Preserved Lemons + Green Olives, page 112), with Korean Slaw (see page 161) and Grilled Corn, Korean Style (see page 158)
Tuesday	Red Smoothie (see page 208)	Lentil Salad with Mustard + Tomatoes (see page 196), Italian Tuna + Chickpea Salad (see page 129), and a pile of arugula	a Bummer Bar (see page 254)	Grilled Duck with Lee's Hoisin Sauce (see page 119) with White Beans, French Style (see page 164) and Roasted Leeks with Shallot Vinaigrette (see page 175)
Wednesday	a Sweet Potato + Five-Spice Muffin (see page 41) with Fresh Ginger Tea (see page 207)	Mr. Chow–Style Minced Chicken with Lettuce Leaves (see page 103)	gluten-free seeded crackers with Pumpkin Seed Pesto (see page 286)	Salmon with Lee's Sriracha + Lime (see page 137), Spicy Brussels Sprouts (see page 154), and Stir-Fried Brown Rice with Nori + Black Sesame (see page 195)
Thursday	Quinoa Granola with Maple Syrup + Olive Oil (see page 30), with almond milk and blueberries	Spanish Chopped Salad with Tuna + Piquillos and Spanish Salad Dressing (see page 66)	Cleo's Afternoon Shake (see page 220)	Super-Crispy Roast Chicken (see page 100), White Bean Puree with Turnip + Roasted Garlic (see page 163), and Broccoli Rabe with Garlic + Red Chili (see page 154)
Friday	Almond + Kale Smoothie (see page 207)	Power Chopped Salad with Creamy Parsley Dressing (see page 61)	a Favorite Baked Apple (see page 266)	Roasted Striped Bass, "Baked Clam" Style (see page 143), with a green salad and boiled new potatoes smashed with goat's milk yogurt, Old Bay seasoning, and chopped fresh chives
Saturday	Poached Eggs with Garlicky Spinach + Crispy Turkey Bacon (see page 38)	Salmon Burgers with Pickled Ginger + Coriander (see page 128) and sautéed snap peas	half an avocado filled with Carrot-Ginger Dressing (see page 65)	Chicken + Turkey Sausage Paella (see page 184) and a nice salad dressed with Spanish Salad Dressing (see page 66)
Sunday	"Buttermilk" Waffles (see page 38)	Easiest Posole (see page 92)	a Millet-Fig Muffin (see page 43)	White Bean + Swiss Chard Soup (see page 82) and Chicken Francese (see page 101) with sautéed spinach

Acknowledgments

Elouisa Rivera
Kevin Keating
Terry Abbott
Georgie Calvocoressi
Oliver Hawthorne
Sonia Tukaj
Lorena Anoch
Victoria Ortiz
Sonia Dumont Lee + Darleen Gross

Food Styling and Production
Susie Theodorou
Molly Shuster

Photography
Ditte Isager
Pippa Drummond
Jonathan Bumble

Prop Styling
Christine Rudolph
Rebecca Bartoshesky
John Miserendino

Art Direction and Design
Erika Oliveira

Grand Central Life & Style
Karen Murgolo
Pippa White
Tareth Mitch
Claire Brown
Jimmy Franco
Peggy Holm
Nicole Bond

• • •

Amber Waves! Katie Baldwin and Amanda Merrow
Charlotte Sasso and all the folks at Stuart's
All the folks at Iacono
All the folks at Ecco Farmstand
Luke Janklow
Stephen Huvane

Index

Conversion Charts

Oven Temperature Equivalents

Degrees Fahrenheit (°F)	Degrees Celcius (°C)	Gas mark
225	110	¼
250	130	½
275	140	1
300	150	2
325	160	3
350	180	4
375	190	5
400	200	6
425	220	7
450	230	8
475	240	9

A quick guide to cup equivalents for liquid

US cups	Metric equivalent	Imperial equivalent
¼ cup	60ml	2fl oz
½ cup	120ml	4fl oz
¾ cup	180ml	6fl oz
1 cup	240ml	8fl oz

About the Authors

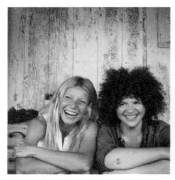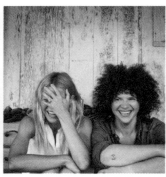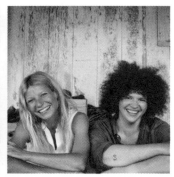

Gwyneth Paltrow is an Oscar winner and author of the *New York Times* bestselling cookbook *My Father's Daughter*, published in the UK as *Notes from my Kitchen Table.* She is a mother and an actress, and splits her time between London and New York. Her website, *GOOP.com*, covers food, travel, fashion, and wellness.

Julia Turshen is a food writer and producer. Most notably, she co-authored *Spain: A Culinary Road Trip* with Mario Batali and *The Kimchi Chronicles* with Marja Vongerichten. Julia's writing has been featured in *Food & Wine* and on the Epicurious website and Gourmet Live blog. Julia lives in New York, where she was born and raised.